I0220344

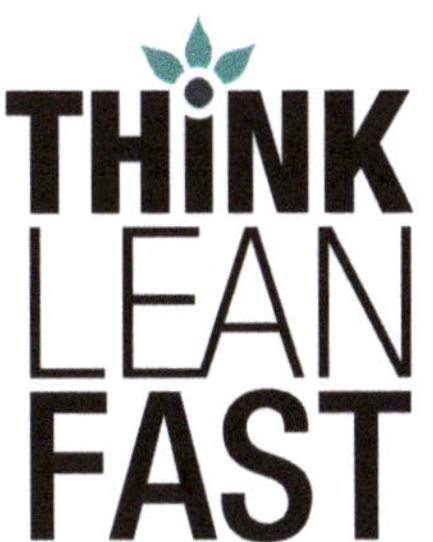
THINK
LEAN
FAST

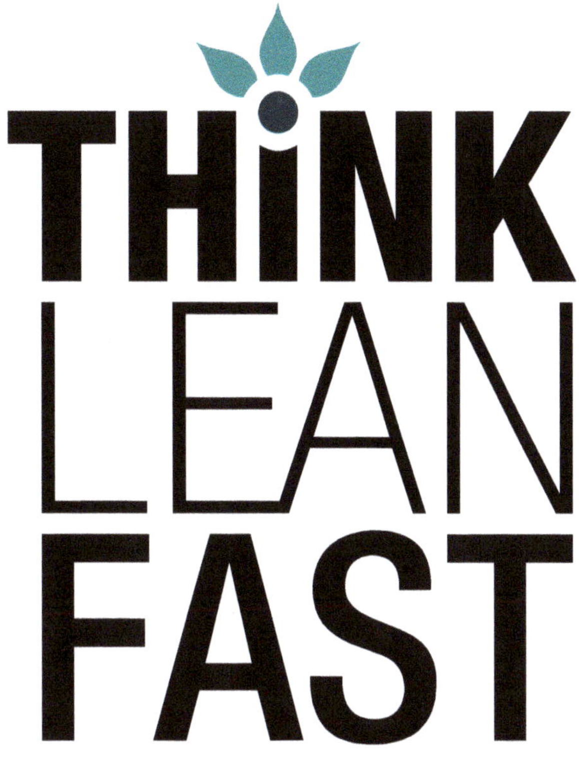

THINK LEAN FAST

HEALTHY LIVING FOR BUSY PEOPLE

Jurie G. **Rossouw**

With Susan D. **Whitmore** and Elle **Cooper**

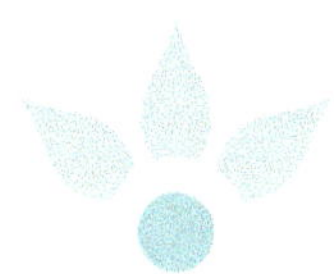

Sydney - Australia

The information in this book is for educational purposes only. It is not intended nor implied to be used as a substitute for professional medical advice. The reader should always consult a healthcare professional to determine the suitability of the information for their own situation or if they have any questions regarding a medical condition or treatment plan. Think Lean Method Pty Ltd, the author and associates are not responsible in any manner whatsoever for any adverse effects directly or indirectly as a result of the information provided in this book.

First printed in 2015

Copyright © Think Lean Method Pty Ltd

All rights reserved. No part of this book may be reproduced or transmitted in any form or by any means whatsoever without express written permission from the author, except in the case of brief quotations embodied in critical articles and reviews. Please refer all pertinent questions to the author.

Jurie G. Rossouw

Susan D. Whitmore

Exercise demonstrations: **Elle Cooper**

Think Lean Method Pty Ltd
PO Box 441
Balgowlah
2093, NSW
Sydney, Australia

ISBN 978-0-99424-121-4

For more information, please contact us through:
www.thinkleanmethod.com

"Life isn't about finding yourself. Life is about creating yourself."

- George Bernard Shaw

Contents

Introduction

"I'm too busy!" "I don't have time!"

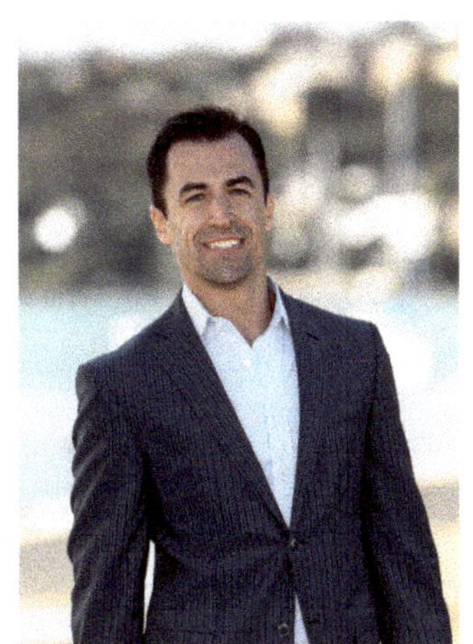

These are two of the most common excuses I hear about why people can't get started with a healthier lifestyle. And to some extent it is true – our lives are increasingly packed full of new activities and responsibilities that seem to consume every last minute we have. As we advance as a civilisation, so it seems that we constantly invent new ways to keep ourselves busy.

Does this necessarily mean the end of a healthy lifestyle filled with nutritious home cooked meals and frequent exercise as we resort to fast foods and instant gratification? Certainly not! Instead, this is our chance to become more productive with how we live a healthy lifestyle and to ***save time*** in the process.

This has been a big theme in my life – I want, *need*, to be healthy, but I still want to have time to work on big personal projects on top of a full time job and still have a social life on the side. The only way to achieve all of this is to focus on faster and simpler ways of doing things. This gives me a ***fast and simple healthy lifestyle*** with the free time I need, while still being healthy and maintaining the body I want. What's more, a healthy body gives me more energy and vitality, meaning I am more productive with the rest of my time. So if there's a way to get much more out of your time and life in general, why not jump at it?

Naturally we want to make sure that a fast healthy lifestyle is based on proven techniques with sound supporting evidence. Many books tell you what worked for one person, but few tell you what has been scientifically proven to work for the broader population. Think Lean Fast follows on from the original Think Lean Method to show you how to achieve a healthy lifestyle based on proven scientific research to create a ***resilient mindset for lasting results***.

Where Think Lean Method goes into all the scientific detail to give you confidence in the method itself, this book builds on those results to gives you a ***quick, easy and versatile guide*** to achieve a healthy lifestyle - fast. The book provides a guide to achieving your goal body, including fast workouts and bulk meals to get you there quickly and save time in the process. It is written in a "choose your own adventure" style, so that you really only need to read the parts that relate to your goals.

You'll find all the tools you need to take charge of your time and get more out of your day. When a healthy lifestyle is this easy to achieve, you'll never allow excuses to hold you back again – ***lasting health and success starts here***!

Jurie G. Rossouw

Start Right, Save Time

1 Start With Your Goals

As a universal rule in life, your actions must support your goals. The fewer actions you take that support your goals, the longer it will take to achieve them. With your body in particular, only through consistently eating the right foods day after day and exercising the right way, can you create the body you want. This is why it is crucial to understand what exactly you want to achieve so that you can determine the right actions to take.

As you get busier and busier, you might just not have the time anymore to cook and also spend an hour in the gym every day. Having your days crammed full of so many activities makes it really difficult to be consistent with a healthy lifestyle so that you actually see the results you want. And, of course, consistency is the one thing that will get you the results you want. Fortunately there have been many advances in nutritional science recently which uncovered simpler and faster ways to achieve your goals.

This gives you a more reliable way to get lean and healthy because *'simple is sustainable'*. The simpler and easier it is for you to reach your body and health goals, the more likely it is that you will stick to it. You'll also be left with more time to do other things, like spending time with friends and family, or perhaps building a career or working on your hobbies. Being more efficient means you don't have to sacrifice as much and you can achieve more in the same amount of time. Of course, this applies to all areas of your life, though for this book we will focus on what to eat and how to exercise.

To get you started, we will now go into more detail about the goal body types and then give you a guide to achieve each of them. These body types are not the usual body shapes that you might be familiar with – instead they are 'goal' body types that anyone can work towards and achieve. In addition to the specific body types, we will also look at another type of goal which aims at simply being healthy and doesn't work towards a specific goal body type.

1.1 Goal body types

What is your vision of your goal body? Is it slim or muscular, lean or curvy, toned or strong? Your vision of your goal body determines what steps you need to take to achieve it. Therefore, it is important that you have a clear vision of your goal body so that you can set the right goals to achieve it.

The three body types we will look at are not genetic and have nothing to do with your height, bone structure, or shapes such as apples or pears. Instead, they are the goal body types that you can achieve regardless of genetics by spending only a few hours a week on nutrition and exercise.

Now, we are all different, so how is this possible?

These body types simply represent different ratios of body fat to muscle mass, which all of us can control through eating and exercise. We'll look at each of the body composition types and the best way to achieve them. There is no right or wrong choice here - it is all up to you which goal body type you prefer. You may already have a vision of your goal body in mind, but it's still worth taking a look at the different body types so you can learn more about composition.

Important!

1. *Remember that your body is unique, so reaching a particular ratio of body fat to muscle mass doesn't mean you'll look exactly like someone else who achieved the same ratio. Focus on the amount of body fat and muscle, rather than the actual body shapes, length of limbs, height etc.* ***You are trying to become the best version of you! Your own unique body is something to value and be proud of!***
2. *A common theme among the goal bodies below is that the body fat levels are usually on the lower end. This is what the Automatic Calorie Management (ACM - explained in detail in Think Lean Method and summarised later in this book) eating guidelines are designed for, providing you with all the nutrients your body needs without the excess energy that gets stored as fat. Just remember - the more free meals you have, the higher your body fat levels will tend to be.*
3. *If you are 30kg to 40kg above where you want to be, skip the workouts, focus on eating healthy to lose weight and just go for a 30 minute walk every other day. Once you have lost the excess weight, you can start training towards your goal body. Eating healthy is the main factor in controlling weight, so you will get results just from eating right!*

1.1.1 Slim / Fashion model look

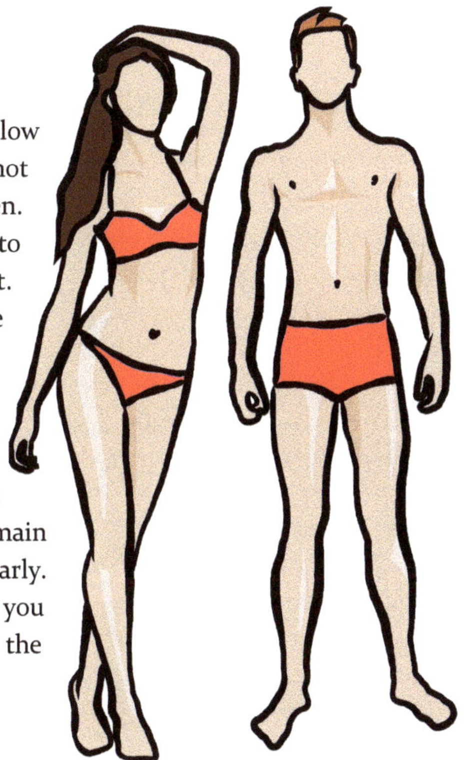

- **Body fat:** Low (15% to 20%)
- **Muscle mass:** Low definition

This is the typical slim / fashion model body type, with both low body fat and muscle mass. This body type is slim and there is not that much muscle to flex, so skin tends to be smooth and even. Keep in mind that few of us have the bone structure and length to actually end up being a fashion model, but that is not important. As I said before, don't worry about trying to look like someone else – you are going to become the best version of you!

It might come as a surprise, but a slim body doesn't require much exercise to achieve due to low levels of muscle mass. If you follow the Core ACM eating guidelines, you can achieve this body type without killing yourself in the gym. Of course, the main challenge is to stick to healthy eating and not indulge too regularly. If you have a hard time losing weight or want faster results, then you will have to incorporate more exercise and move up to the Advanced Level.

1.1.2 Lean / Bikini body

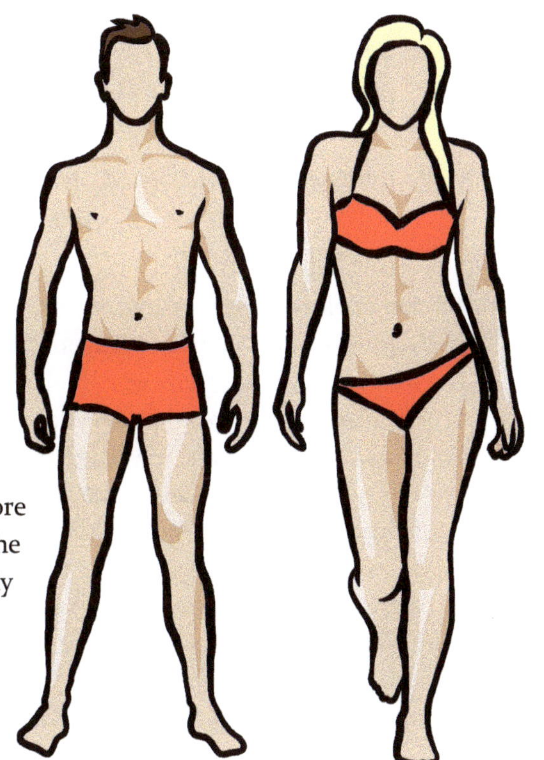

- **Body fat:** Low (15% to 20%)
- **Muscle mass:** Some to good definition

Long a favourite of guys who don't want to get too muscular, going lean has been gaining momentum among females as it can create a strong yet feminine look. With this body type, you get a bit of muscle to flex with some decent curves around the rear and legs. Overall, being 'lean' is a tight and toned look, often referred to as the bikini model look.

Lean bodies have more muscle, which means spending a bit more time exercising. This is great because it means you'll enjoy the metabolic and brain boosting effects as you watch your body change. Overall, this is a very healthy body type!

1.1.3 Athletic / Fitness model look

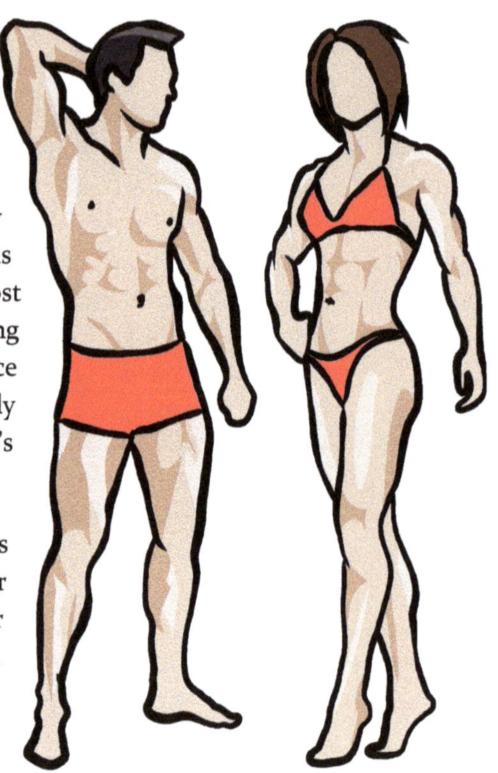

- **Body fat:** Low to very low (12% to 20% for females, 8% to 15% for males)
- **Muscle mass:** Good to great muscle definition

Athletic looking bodies are achieved by increasing muscle mass and definition. You'll have some decent biceps to show off and defined, shapely thighs. You'll see most fitness models and female competitors with this body type. While most females tend to go for the Slim or Lean look, there is a growing interest in getting athletic bodies. This is also a common choice for men and is usually the one I personally go for, mainly because it's easy to maintain, doesn't take much time and it's great for health.

Athletic bodies have a more muscle mass, which means prioritising time to exercise. You'll also need to increase your food intake, so a few extra meals a day is the perfect plan for this. Working out and building muscle is great for your overall health, and as with the Lean body type, you'll get the metabolic and brain boosting effects of regular exercise.

1.1.4 Bodybuilder

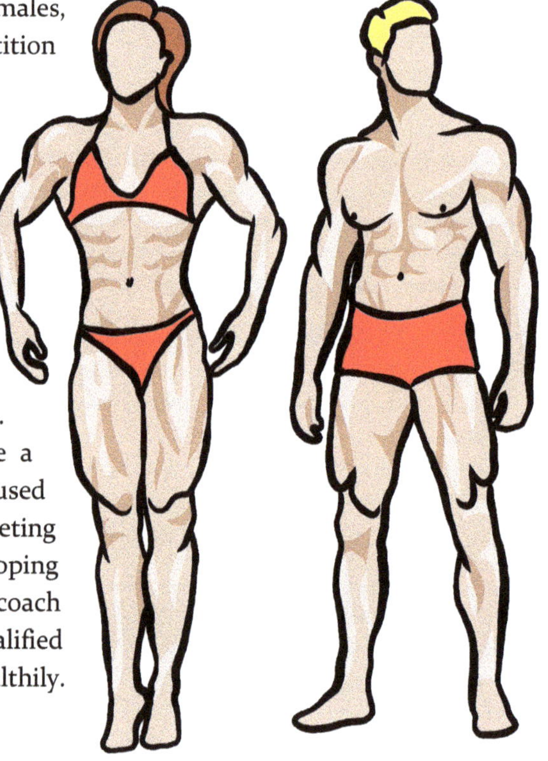

- **Body fat:** Medium off season (20% to 25% for females, 10% to 15% for males). Very low during competition prep (8% to 12% for females, 5% to 7% for males).
- **Muscle mass:** Great to extreme muscle definition (depending if you are on a bulking or cutting cycle)

In this book we are focusing on the previous three body types – Slim, Lean, and Athletic. However there is a fourth body type that is worth calling out, and that is the bodybuilder type. Bodybuilders have extreme amounts of muscle mass, way more than the other types. It takes a huge amount of time and effort to become a bodybuilder, so we won't cover it here as this book is focused on fast workouts and meals. If you are interested in competing in bodybuilding competitions or are serious about developing a lot of muscle, then I strongly recommend you get a coach that is an ex-champion bodybuilder. They will be best qualified to help you reach your body goals safely and healthily.

1.2 Achieving your goal body

Now let's set out a plan to achieve your goal body! From here it's all about taking the right actions to achieve your goal. The way we do this is simple - each body type is shown in the table below along with eating and exercise plans to follow. Since all of our bodies are a bit different, the eating plans depend on how easily you manage weight. Some people are naturally more muscular, some naturally slimmer, and some naturally put on weight faster. These are aspects to be aware of and account for, so that you can maximise success.

Really take a moment to think about what you want to achieve. Why? Because so often we want what we don't have and we ignore what we could more easily achieve. For example, if you put on weight easily but you want to achieve a slim body, then you'll need to work out and stay very clean with your diet. But on the other hand, putting on weight easily means you will gain muscle easier than other people, which in turn means you'll get better results if you start doing heavier weights. Instead of working really hard to keep weight down, you can embrace your body type and more easily build an athletic body instead. Remember - it is easier to work with your body, rather than against it!

1.2.1 Nutrition plans – The three food pyramids

Throughout this book we will be referencing three food pyramids that are specifically designed to give you the right nutritional approach to reach your goals. These food pyramids also give you the flexibility to move between plans if you want to try a different approach or if your goals change. The key is that there is no one right way for everyone – it all depends on what you want to achieve!

Each food pyramid has a name to make it easier to refer to throughout the book. Let's look at all three now:

- ***Think Lean Pyramid*** – this is the main food pyramid that we established in the original Think Lean Method. It is flexible and takes advantage of the latest nutritional neuroscience advances to be an easy and effective way to manage weight and stay healthy in the long term. This is great for weight loss and works through Automatic Calorie Management (ACM) so that you don't have to count calories anymore
- ***Think Free Pyramid*** – if you are good with self-discipline, this food pyramid includes more variety of foods, giving you more freedom to eat what you want
- ***Think Big Pyramid*** – for those looking to get more muscle mass or who have trouble gaining weight, this is the food pyramid for you. Be prepared to eat a lot!

Use the *Goal Body Matrix* below to determine which food pyramid is right for you. To be clear, the idea is not to start with one and then progress through to the others – instead, pick the one that suits you and stick to it!

1.2.2 The goal body matrix

This is your tool to find out what to eat, how many meals to eat per day, and what exercises to do. To use the table, do the following:

1. Find your goal body in the table below using the definitions we covered above, or pick the last column if you are after overall health, regardless of body type

2. Consider how easily you tend to lose weight. Do you find the weight comes off easily when you try (or maybe you actually find it hard to put weight on), is it a massive struggle and the weight never seems to come off, or are you somewhere in-between?
3. Use the combination of your goal body and how easily you lose weight to locate which food pyramid is right for you. Where there is a choice of meal plan, I recommend starting with the one in bold. However, if you feel you are very disciplined and can handle a bit more freedom, you can try the ***Think Free Pyramid*** where indicated
4. Check the matrix to see how many meals to eat per day. Increasing the number of meals isn't going to increase or decrease your metabolism (we busted that myth in *Think Lean Method*), and makes it easier for you to get all the nutrients you need to reach your goal body
5. Choose from the recommended exercise programs. There are Main and Advanced Levels of exercises, depending on your appetite for working out and the kind of results you want to achieve. Obviously if you want faster results, go for Advanced. If you are a beginner, start with the Main Level which should be enough to get results!

The Goal Body Matrix

		Slim Fashion model	**Lean** Bikini body	**Athletic** Fitness model look	**Just want to be healthy**
	Muscle definition	Low definition	Some definition	Good definition	-
	Body fat	Low	Low	Low to very low	-
Nutrition - How easily do you lose weight?	**Hard**	***Think Lean Pyramid - Core ACM*** One free meal p/w	***Think Lean Pyramid - Core ACM*** One free meal p/w	***Think Lean Pyramid - Complete ACM*** (Or Think Free Pyramid) One free meal p/w	***Think Lean Pyramid - Core ACM*** One free meal p/w
	In-between	***Think Lean Pyramid - Core ACM*** One free meal p/w	***Think Lean Pyramid - Complete ACM*** (Or Think Free Pyramid) One free meal p/w	***Think Lean Pyramid - Complete ACM*** (Or Think Free Pyramid) One free meal p/w	***Think Lean Pyramid - Core ACM*** (Or Think Free Pyramid) One free meal p/w
	Easily	***Think Lean Pyramid - Complete ACM*** (Or Think Free Pyramid) One free meal p/w	***Think Lean Pyramid - Complete ACM*** (Or Think Free Pyramid) One free meal p/w	***Think Big Pyramid - Intermittent Carb Cycling*** One free meal p/w	***Think Lean Pyramid - Complete ACM*** (Or Think Free Pyramid) One free meal p/w
	Meals per day	**3 meals p/day**	**3 meals p/day**	**4 - 5 meals p/day**	**3 meals p/day**
Exercise	**Main level**	Stay active, go for walks	***Body HIIT*** or ***Lean HIIT*** workouts four times a week	***Heavy HIIT*** workouts four times a week	Do whatever exercise or activities you enjoy
	Advanced level (addition to Main level)	***Pure HIIT*** or ***Body HIIT*** workouts 3 or more times per week	***Pure HIIT*** on two days and ***Lean HIIT on*** four days (six days total per week)	For lower body fat, add two to four ***Pure HIIT*** sessions per week	***Pure HIIT*** or ***Body HIIT*** workouts 3 or more times per week.
	Overall time investment	**2 - 3 hours p/week**	**3 - 4 hours p/week**	**3 - 5 hours p/week**	**2 - 3 hours p/week**

In the last row you can see the estimated **overall time investment** needed in a week to achieve your goal body. This includes both meal preparation and workouts. The plans in this book will help you achieve your goal body in the most efficient way. Of course, you can add in more variety, though that might need a bit more time investment from you. The Main Level workouts are faster than the Advanced Level, so if you are following the Advanced Level you might need a bit more time each week. Overall, most of these plans are possible to follow in around three hours a week.

Wait - three hours a week? That's just over 25 minutes per day! Considering that a lot of people spend an hour in the gym nearly every day, then many more hours a week cooking meals, this is a massive time saving! You get hours back in your day to spend on the things important to you *and still get the body you want*!

1.2.3 What are the 'free meals'?

Each meal plan includes one free meal per week. This is for you to enjoy eating whatever you like, and you can fit the free meal in whenever you prefer. Just remember that if you want to include more free meals per week, your body fat levels will end up being higher than the target bodies above. Is this bad? Not necessarily! A lean or athletic body type with a bit of extra body fat will simply make you curvy, which can be attractive on both females and males! As long as you are healthy, happy and confident with the body you have, then all is well.

A note on strategies for free meals – if your free meal is a huge bowl of ice cream, large pizza or other food type that's both high in carbohydrates and dietary fat, you will slow down progress towards achieving your goal body. I tend to gear my free meals towards something that is still high in protein, like a nice big steak. If you do want some ice cream or sugary snacks, try to savour each bite and have a bit less than usual. The next bite will be just as good as the current one, so enjoy the bite you're with! This way you are always practicing portion control.

1.3 Get started!

Have you got a clear vision of your target goal body? Great! Have you picked one of the options above with meal and exercise plans to achieve it? Fantastic! You can write these down in the Think Lean Tracking Sheet at the end of this book and get started!

In the **Personal Vision** section, write down the target body type that is your goal. As we mentioned in *Think Lean Method* – make the statement future-oriented and talk as if you have it already. This helps motivate you for better results. For example, "I *have* a lean body".

In the **Prioritised Goals** section, write down two clear goals – one for your eating plan and one for you exercise plan. For example:

- "I will do Lean HIIT workouts four times a week for the next three months, starting [today's date]"
- "I will follow Complete ACM with only one free meal per week for the next three months, starting [today's date]"

Remember to prioritise them against your other life goals. If your vision is hugely important to you, put it high up. If you have some other important commitments, put it after those.

Now it is time to start building your goal body to make that vision a reality. Up next – nutrition!

Nutrition First

2 Nutrition Plans

What you eat is by far the most important element of achieving the body you want. Each meal either moves you towards or away from your goal. Building your goal body and level of health means you need to stay consistent with the right nutrition plan, and when it comes to consistency, there is one rule that is absolutely key – simple is sustainable! Keeping your meals and preparation simple means it is easier to stick to it day after day.

Nutrition plans in this section focus on ways to keep everything fast and efficient to give you time back in your day. In a way, you will learn how to become your own healthy fast food vendor or favourite take away shop. The meal plans are the starting point, providing you with fast and nutritious recipes which you can start to modify if you want to add in more variety. For some people, variety is very important so they are willing to invest the additional time. Others, like me, really value the time savings from sticking to simple meal plans. Personally, I have a lot of other things that keep me busy, so I'm happy to have less fancy meals so I can get time back for the more important stuff.

I recommend that you start with a simple meal plan and then modify from there as you like. The meal plans are explained through the food pyramids, which are designed to support you to reach your goals. To get started, use the name of the food pyramid from the goal matrix along with the number of meals.

Note - These plans are not all-or-nothing!

Following these meal plans does not mean you have to give up your favourite foods forever. The reality is that you can still get most of the benefits even if you don't follow the meal plans 100% of the time. I include one "free meal" per week in the meal plans below as standard. Free meals are different from cheat meals since they are part of the plan. For example, you can have your free meal any time you like during the week, but if you have another one, it would be a cheat meal because it wasn't part of your plan.

Basic nutrition rules

After a great deal of research which I wrote about in Think Lean Method, I've distilled good nutrition down to five simple rules. These rules give you high-level guidelines to follow to manage weight, stay healthy and reach your goals:

1. **Quality protein with every meal** – The main satiating factor in meals is protein, which is also the least fattening. Protein helps to improve lean muscle mass which keeps your metabolism high. This is why we want to include quality protein with every meal. Preferable sources are meats and eggs as they provide high quality protein with all amino acids and high bioavailability.
2. **Low-GI carbohydrates** – These are used differently in the three food pyramids to help you reach your goals:
    - ***Think Lean Pyramid*** – cut out sugars and grains for a total nutritional transformation. This helps you lose weight without counting calories
    - ***Think Free Pyramid*** – add in wholegrain foods and a bit of sugar to give you more freedom, provided you stick to the portion sizes
    - ***Think Big Pyramid*** – includes lots of whole grain foods to help fuel muscle growth

   Remember, high-GI carbohydrate foods such as sugars, refined grains and processed foods are the main culprits that make you gain weight and affect your health!
3. **Whole foods** – Sticking to whole, unprocessed foods is one of the simplest ways to cut down on fattening foods. Foods like breads, pasta, salami, sweets and so on are all processed foods. The more processed they are, the faster they are absorbed and the more body fat they add!
4. **Mix it up** – This is a cardinal rule to prevent slow overdoses or deficiencies of vitamins and minerals. Switch around your meals from time to time and vary your recipes. This will not just keep you healthy, but it will also keep it interesting!
5. **Slow down** – In Think Lean Method we talk about the neurotransmitters that help you feel full, but they need time to work! Slow down the speed you eat at so that you allow yourself enough time to actually feel full. And stop eating when you are full!

Meal plan templates

This book provides you with guidelines to help you build a plan that suits your lifestyle. To help with this and provide extra flexibility for you to build your own plans, you'll see icons in the meal plan templates for you to match up with the recipes, or even to cook up your own meals that suit the plans.

All you have to do is check the icons in the meal plans and match them to the icons in the recipes to see which ingredients to use. This also means you can use each of the recipes in many different ways by varying the ingredients. Simple yet flexible!

The food icons (explained on the next page) are for the main food groups, focusing on different types of proteins (lean meats and fatty meats) and carbohydrates (low-GI, starchy vegetables, and wholegrain). In Think Lean Method we explained that eating the right kind of macronutrients are important for different types of goals, so this is all designed to get you the body you want!

Protein sources

Lean Meats

Lean meats usually have 5% or less dietary fat, and have no or very little visible strips of fat in the meat. Be sure to trim any visible fat prior to cooking if there is any, since cooking fat will seep into the rest of the meat.

Examples:
- Chicken breast
- Sirloin
- Tenderloin
- Round steak
- 95% lean ground beef
- Fish (leave the skin on)

Fatty Meats

Fatty meats have visible strips of dietary fat and are the more marbled cuts of meat. They provide more energy than lean meats, making them ideal for when you are working out a lot.

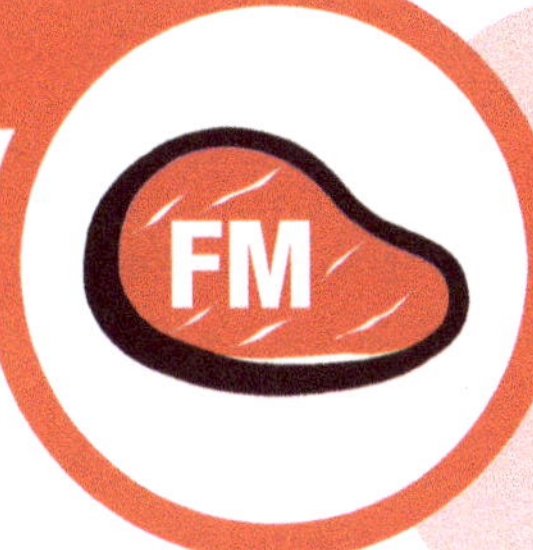

Examples:
- Chicken thighs
- Porterhouse steak
- Ribeye steak
- T-bone steak
- Wagyu
- Ribs
- Lamb
- Pork

Carbohydrate sources

Low-GI Vegetables

You can eat a large amount of these vegetables without having to worry about calories, so really they are free foods! They are packed with nutrients and super healthy, so add in a few extra servings.

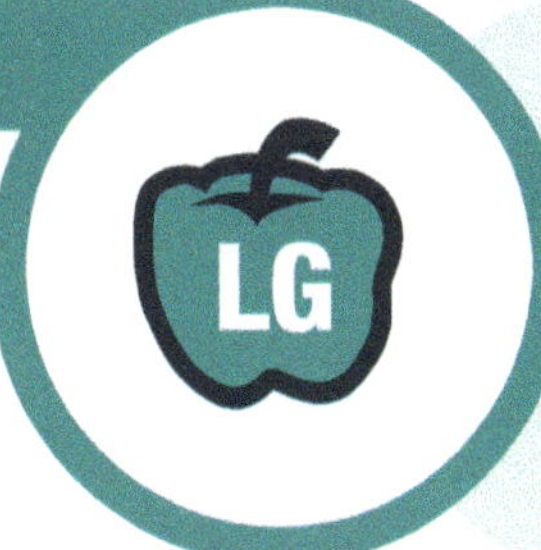

Examples:
- Asparagus
- Broccoli
- Cabbage
- Carrots
- Cucumber
- Lettuce
- Mushrooms
- Onions
- Peppers
- Spinach
- Squash
- Tomatoes
- Zucchini

Starchy Vegetables

These vegetables are more calorie-dense, so pair them with the right foods to get the best out of them. Even though legumes are not technically vegetables, we include them here since they are a rich source of carbohydrates.

Examples:
- Beets
- Chickpeas
- Green peas
- Kidney beans
- Lentils
- Plantains
- Pumpkin
- Sweet corn
- Sweet potato
- Yams

Whole Grains

Much higher in carbohydrates than vegetables, whole grain foods are useful for when you are working out a lot and want to build an athletic body. Try to eat whole grains (not refined) and go for lower-GI grain foods.

Examples:
- Rolled oats
- Brown rice
- Barley
- Quinoa
- Buckwheat
- Semolina

Stick to whole foods, but these can work if you control portions sizes:
- Wholewheat pasta
- Wholewheat bread
- Sourdough
- Rye bread

2.1 Think Lean Pyramid – Automatic Calorie Management

The ***Think Lean Pyramid*** is based on an extensive review of nutrition and neuroscience research I completed. It includes an effect that I call Automatic Calorie Management (ACM). The great thing about this pyramid is that it provides full nutrition for a healthy body and brain, while taking advantage of neuroscience advances so you can eat large meals that make you feel full while still getting the body you want. If you'd like more detail on the scientific basis of the ***Think Lean Pyramid***, refer to the original Think Lean Method book.

2.1.1 What it works for

ACM is all about managing your caloric intake automatically. This makes it particularly useful if you have trouble stopping eating when you are full, as with ACM you can eat large meals without having to worry about putting on weight.

Personally, I used to be a big sugar fiend - nougat and sugary drinks every single day. Chocolates too, but mostly high-sugar sweets. Now it is all different. Switching to ACM has resulted in me totally giving up sugars without missing them at all. This is because of a neuroscience principle that says "neurons that fire apart, wire apart". What this means is that cutting out sugars and changing how you think about them changes your brain and breaks down those unhelpful neural pathways that cause cravings. This has really worked for me - even a big slice of cake or nougat in front of my mouth does not cause me to crave it anymore. It's amazing! Instead I crave being healthy and keeping the body I want.

Think Lean can change your brain and is part of a larger Mental Fitness framework. In particular, ACM is great for:

- If you are looking for a simple and practical way to be healthy
- If you have a hard time controlling your appetite
- If you are exercising a lot and want to keep/build lean muscle
- If you are not actively exercising but still want to lose weight

Note that the ***Think Lean Pyramid*** mainly helps for losing body fat and getting lean, and therefore is not ideal for bulking up. By its very nature it will cause you to feel full before you get enough nutrients for huge muscle growth, since it automatically manages your caloric intake to be fairly low.

Still, this food pyramid can be adapted to your lifestyle and your goal, so it is highly versatile. It is great for slim and lean bodies, and can even be used to get athletic by increasing the number of meals a day. The goal body matrix shows you which version of ACM to use and how many meals to fit in per day to get to your goal body.

2.1.2 Why it works

The concept of ACM is that by eating the right food groups, you simply don't have to count calories. These foods keep you lean and healthy, and are also great for your brain. We can get so focused on our bodies that we tend to forget that without a healthy brain, we won't have the energy or willpower to stick to a healthy eating lifestyle! With ACM, nutritional neuroscience and neuropsychotherapy comes together to make you healthy, lean and confident. This is how it works:

- **Controls your appetite.** Nutritional neuroscience research shows that protein[1,2] and dietary fats[3] are the best at making you feel full. By adding more protein into meals, you feel full faster and stay full for longer. This controls your appetite to reduce snacking and keeps you lean. At first glance it might look like this contains too much protein, however in *Think Lean Method* we bust the myths around excess protein (see Think Lean Method section 2.4.4) and go into detail about the benefits for getting lean and being healthy.
- **Burns more calories.** Research on metabolism shows that a diet higher in protein helps you burn more calories since you retain more muscle mass as you lose weight[4]. This means you keep a higher metabolism when compared to high-carb, low-protein diets. In addition, the body burns 30% of the caloric value of protein to digest it[5]. This effectively means that 100g of carbohydrates is equivalent to around 140g of protein, making protein a fantastic and filling weight-loss component of your diet!
- **Adds nutritious food.** By upping your intake of vegetables as an awesome source of nutrients and low-GI carbohydrates, you eat large, filling meals while still giving the body a chance to burn fat. New research also shows that eating lots of vegetables every day helps people live longer[6]! ACM limits foods with omega-6, meaning you reduce systemic inflammation and improve your overall health. We also need other nutrients, which is why we include dairy products, meat and nuts for a complete, healthy diet. Of course this includes all the herbs and spices you want!
- **Provides consistent energy.** By skipping high-GI and calorie-dense foods like grains and sugar, we get consistent energy and get off the rollercoaster of blood sugar spikes and crashes. Sugar and high-GI carbohydrates cause serotonin to release in your brain and have addictive properties[7,8], but once you cut them from your diet, the neural networks that cause your cravings will start to dissipate and you will not even miss them!

If you'd like more information, ACM and this food pyramid is fully explained in *Think Lean Method* with all rules defined in detail, including citations of over a hundred studies.

2.1.3 Guidelines

In the diagram below you'll see the ***Think Lean Pyramid*** is split into two sections depending on the amount of exercise you do.

- **Core ACM** where you can eat as much as you like of specific food groups and lose weight, even with little or no exercise (excludes legumes, starchy vegetables and fatty meats)
- **Complete ACM** where you can eat as much as you like from a wider group of foods provided you are living an active lifestyle with regular gym/exercise sessions each week (includes legumes, starchy vegetables and fatty meats for extra energy and workout recovery)

From here onwards follow the plan that you selected in the Goal Body Matrix.

The size of the segments in the pyramid indicates the relative number of calories you get from each food group. All of this will be taken care of by using the recipes so don't worry about any calorie counting.

Note – Just because Core ACM is smaller than Complete ACM on the pyramid doesn't mean you should physically eat less. You can still eat the same amount of food as before, what is important is the type of foods you eat, which is what the Core ACM section shows you. Use the meal plans below to see how much to eat with each meal. You can think of Core ACM and Complete ACM as two sides of the pyramid:

- If you need to lose weight and keep it off with little exercise, or if you find it really hard to lose weight and keep it off, stay focused on the Core ACM side of the pyramid
- If you need more calories to support you working out a lot, then you can look at both sides of the pyramid

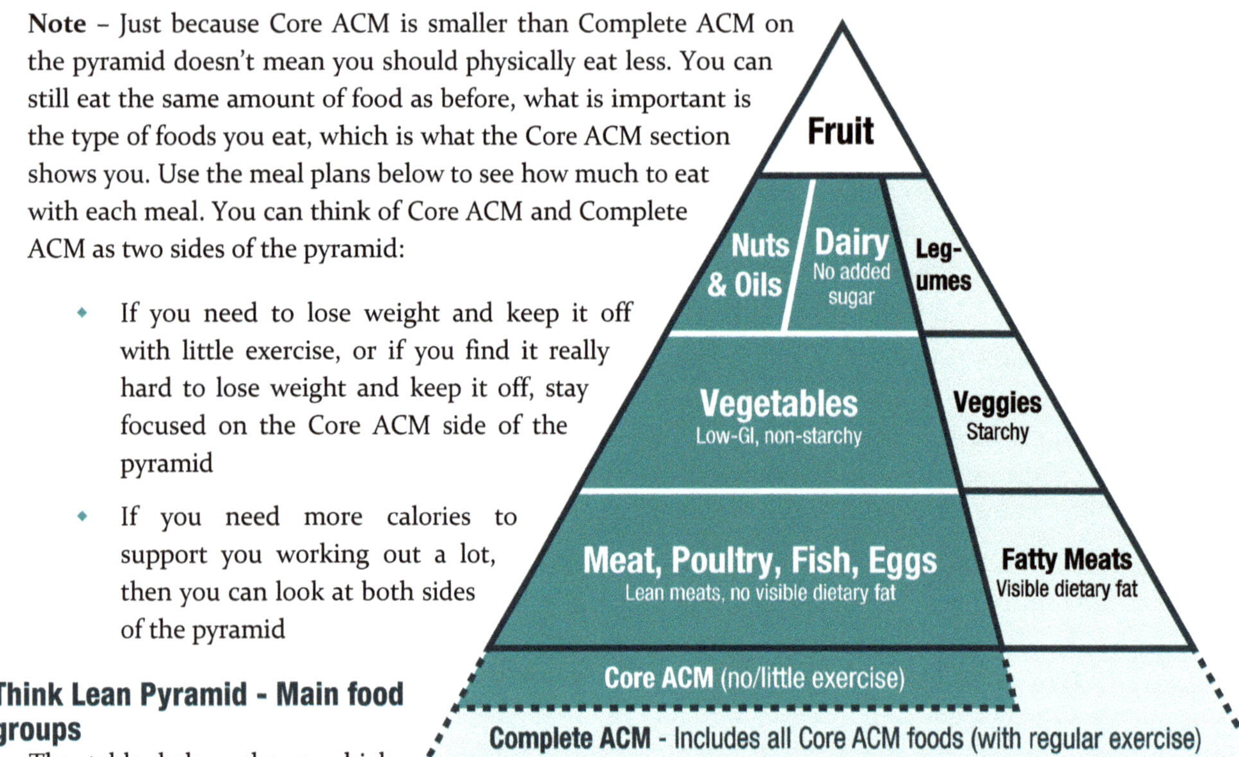

Think Lean Pyramid - Main food groups

The table below shows which foods are generally in or out and how much to eat at a time. These give a general indication, however the exact amounts you'll eat would vary depending on your goal, so use the meal plans provided to work out how much exactly to eat. ***Also, see the end of the book for full food lists for this food pyramid.***

Food type	Core ACM	Complete ACM	Portions	Notes
Lean meats & eggs	Yes	Yes	Two servings for a meal.	Eat most of to build muscle and stay full throughout the day. LM
Fatty meats	No	Yes	Two servings for a meal.	If following Complete ACM, eat with every third meal. Preferably eat with low-GI carbohydrates. FM
Low-GI vegetables	Yes	Yes	Three servings for a meal.	Eat as much as you want! The more, the better. LG
Starchy vegetables	No	Yes	Two to three servings for a meal.	Include as one of every three meals for Complete ACM and eat with lean protein sources. SV
Nuts	Yes	Yes	One serving per day.	Use as snacks or to garnish meals.
Oils	Yes	Yes	Use oils sparingly.	Coconut oil works best as it is low in omega-6. Sunflower and most other plant oils are high in omega-6, so try to limit these. Butter is an alternative for cooking. Extra virgin olive oil is also a better choice than other plant oils.
Dairy	Yes	Yes	One serving per day.	Unsweetened dairy products are a good addition as they are the primary source of calcium in our diets. If you can't tolerate dairy, consider taking a Calcium supplement.
Legumes	No	Yes	One serving per day.	Since they are often higher on the glycaemic index, they are reserved for Complete ACM.
Fruit	Yes	Yes	One serving or one piece of fruit a day.	Just because they are at the top doesn't mean they are bad! The other foods sources are simply better for us than fruits, due to the high sugar content of fruits.

Think Lean Pyramid - Other foods

This table lists other common foods you might be wondering about. Some are good (green), some should be limited (grey), and some are out (red). Foods in red can be eaten as part of the weekly free meal, though try to keep the free meal to a reasonable size!

Food type	Core ACM	Complete ACM	Notes
Water	Yes	Yes	Make this your drink of choice! Drink more to help you feel full.
Herbs & spices	Yes	Yes	Eat as much as you like! This is a great way to spice up foods in a guilt-free way.
Sweeteners	Yes	Yes	Generally try to cut out sweet foods, but if you really want something sweet, try a natural sweetener like xylitol, stevia or erythritol. Chewing gum and sweets that use sweeteners are fine.
Caffeine	Limit	Limit	Stick to one cup of coffee per day, preferably at the start of the day.
Alcohol	Limit	Limit	White wines and champagne are often better choices. Cut out cocktails and mixers as they are high in sugars. Try to keep to just one or two glasses a week.
Grains	No	No	ACM is a grain-free eating plan since grains encourage you to overeat and are high in Omega-6. Cut out grains to make weight management easy and keep you healthy! WG
Sugar, sweets, soft drinks, etc.	No	No	Go sugar free! Cut out any foods with added sugar.
Chocolate	No	No	Most types contain sugar and are highly processed, so limit these to free meals. Sugar free chocolate is something you can enjoy more regularly.

2.1.4 Meal plan templates

By now you should know which side of ACM you are going with and how many meals to eat per day. Find the right combination below and use this as your starting meal plan. Of course, these plans are all focused on being highly efficient so you spend less time cooking. I recommend starting with the meal plan as is, then modify from there to suit your lifestyle and tastes.

These plans are set up as **templates**, so they show you what kinds of foods to eat with each meal, along with a suggestion for each. You can use these to experiment with different recipes while still sticking to the overall plan, allowing you to easily create your own meal plans. The full *Think Lean Method* contains heaps more healthy recipes you can fit in if you prefer more variety.

While we're on the topic, a note on variety - If you absolutely cannot stand the thought of eating the same thing for a few days in a row, then here is a simple solution - spend one Sunday each month cooking up a bunch of meals, divide them up for the month, freeze, then pick out what you feel like each day. This way you get loads of variety and have a whole month free of cooking! Otherwise you can keep breakfast and lunch the same, and vary diner each day. The only limitation is your own creativity. The options are endless!

Think Lean Core ACM: ***3-Meal Plan Template***

- Do your meal prep on Sundays. Eat one portion and save the rest for the week days
- On Saturdays you can have other meals, though stick to eating the right food groups for two of the three meals at least
- For **variety**, try cooking more recipes on Sunday so that you can eat different meals through the week. Otherwise you can skip the dinner meal prep and making something different each night
- Use fruit and nuts for snacks

	Breakfast	Lunch	Dinner
Sunday to Friday	LM + LG Prepare a **Fast Frittata (page 36)** for the week – 15 mins. Eat one portion and store rest for the week	LM + LG Prepare a **Fast Chicken Bake (page 48)** – 10 mins. Eat one portion and store rest for the week	LM + LG Prepare **Chilli Con Sus (page 44)** – 25 mins. Eat one portion and store rest for the week
Saturday	LM + LG 3 egg omelette with mushrooms, spinach and tomato	LM + LG BBQ Steak with steamed vegetables	FREE *Free meal! Eat what you like, but try to control portion sizes*
Sunday to Friday	LM + LG Prepare **Almond Pancakes (page 38)** for the week – 15 mins. Eat one portion and store rest for the week	LM + LG Prepare a **Beef Stew (page 50)** – 20 mins. Eat one portion and store rest for the week	LM + LG Prepare a **Lamb Roast (page 52)** – 10 mins. Eat one portion and store rest for the week
Saturday	LM + LG Protein smoothie with coconut water, carrots and peaches	LM + LG Chicken breast with lemon, cumin, paprika and pepper. Add cauliflower rice	FREE *Free meal! Eat what you like, but try to control portion sizes*
Sunday to Friday	LM + LG Prepare **Omega Quiche Muffins (page 40)** for the week – 20 mins. Eat one portion and store rest for the week	LM + LG Prepare **Turkey Burgers (page 46)** – 20 mins. Eat one portion and store rest for the week	LM + LG Prepare **Fish Galore (page 57)** – 10 mins. Eat one portion and store rest for the week
Saturday	LM + LG 3 egg omelette with mushrooms, spinach and tomato	LM + LG Grilled salmon with steamed vegetables	FREE *Free meal! Eat what you like, but try to control portion sizes*

Think Lean Complete ACM: 3-Meal Plan Template

- Do your meal prep on Sundays. Eat one portion and save the rest for the week days
- On Saturdays you can have other meals, though stick to eating the right food groups for two of the three meals at least
- For **variety**, try cooking more recipes on Sunday so that you can eat different meals through the week. Otherwise you can skip the dinner meal prep and make something different each night
- Use fruit and nuts for snacks

	Breakfast	Lunch	Dinner
Sunday to Friday	LM + SV Prepare a **Fast Frittata (page 36)** for the week – 15 mins. Eat one portion and store rest for the week	LM + LG Prepare a **Fast Chicken Bake (page 48)** – 10 mins. Eat one portion and store rest for the week	FM + LG Prepare **Chilli Con Sus (page 44)** – 25 mins. Eat one portion and store rest for the week
Saturday	LM + LG 3 egg omelette with mushrooms, spinach and tomato	FM + LG BBQ Steak with steamed vegetables	FREE *Free meal! Eat what you like, but try to control portion sizes*
Sunday to Friday	LM + LG Prepare **Omega Quiche Muffins (page 40)** for the week – 15 mins. Eat one portion and store rest for the week	LM + SV Prepare **Anytime Meatballs (page 54)** – 10 mins. Eat one portion and store rest for the week	FM + LG Prepare a **Lamb Roast (page 52)** – 10 mins. Eat one portion and store rest for the week
Saturday	LM + LG Sugar-free yoghurt with mix berries and crushed nuts	FM + LG Chicken thigh with lemon, cumin, paprika and pepper. Add cauliflower rice	FREE *Free meal! Eat what you like, but try to control portion sizes*
Sunday to Friday	LM + LG Prepare **Almond Bread (page 42)** for the week – 15 mins. Eat one portion and store rest for the week	LM + SV Prepare **Turkey Burgers (page 46)** – 20 mins. Eat one portion and store rest for the week	FM + LG Prepare a **Beef Stew (page 50)** – 25 mins. Eat one portion and store rest for the week
Saturday	FM + LG 3 scrambled eggs with 2 strips of bacon, sautéed mushrooms and tomato	LM + LG Grilled salmon with steamed vegetables	FREE *Free meal! Eat what you like, but try to control portion sizes*

*Think Lean Complete ACM: **4-Meal Plan Template***

- Do your meal prep on Sundays. Eat one portion and save the rest for the week days
- On Saturdays you can have other meals, though stick to eating the right food groups for two of the three meals at least
- Use fruit and nuts for snacks
- **Speed it up** by replacing Lunch 1 or Lunch 2 with a protein shake or smoothie

	Breakfast	Lunch 1	Lunch 2	Dinner
Sunday to Friday	LM + SV Prepare a **Fast Frittata (page 36)** for the week – 15 mins. Eat one portion and store rest for the week	LM + LG Prepare a **Fast Chicken Bake (page 48)** – 10 mins. Eat one portion and store rest for the week	LM + LG Prepare a **Bulk Bolognese (page)** – 10 mins. Eat one portion and store rest for the week	FM + LG Prepare **Chilli Con Sus (page 44)** – 25 mins. Eat one portion and store rest for the week
Saturday	LM + LG 3 egg omelette with mushrooms, spinach and tomato	FM + LG BBQ Steak with steamed vegetables	LM + LG Grilled salmon with steamed vegetables	FREE *Free meal! Eat what you like, but try to control portion sizes*
Sunday to Friday	LM + LG Prepare **Omega Quiche Muffins (page 40)** for the week – 15 mins. Eat one portion and store rest for the week	LM + SV Prepare **Anytime Meatballs (page 54)** – 10 mins. Eat one portion and store rest for the week	LM + LG Prepare **Fish Galore (page 57)** – 10 mins. Eat one portion and store rest for the week	FM + LG Prepare a **Lamb Roast (page 52)** – 10 mins. Eat one portion and store rest for the week
Saturday	LM + LG Sugar-free yoghurt with mix berries and crushed nuts	LM + LG Chicken breast with lemon, cumin, paprika and pepper. Add cauliflower rice	FM + LG Lamb cooked with sage and spinach, steamed vegetables on the side	FREE *Free meal! Eat what you like, but try to control portion sizes*
Sunday to Friday	LM + LG Prepare **Almond Bread (page 42)** for the week – 15 mins. Eat one portion and store rest for the week	LM + LG Prepare **Turkey Burgers (page 46)** – 20 mins. Eat one portion and store rest for the week	LM + SV Prepare **Fast Chicken Bake (page 48)** – 10 mins. Eat one portion and store rest for the week	FM + LG Prepare a **Beef Stew (page 50)** – 25 mins. Eat one portion and store rest for the week
Saturday	FM + LG 3 scrambled eggs with 2 strips of bacon, sautéed mushrooms and tomato	LM + LG Grilled salmon with steamed vegetables	LM + LG Chicken breast with roast capsicum, mushrooms, oregano and thyme	FREE *Free meal! Eat what you like, but try to control portion sizes*

*Think Lean Complete ACM: **5-Meal Plan Template***

- Do your meal prep on Sundays. Eat one portion and save the rest for the week days
- On Saturdays you can have other meals, though stick to eating the right food groups for two of the three meals at least
- For **variety**, try cooking more recipes on Sunday so that you can eat different meals through the week. Otherwise you can skip the dinner meal prep and make something different each night
- To **speed things up**, try making a double amount of each recipe so you can cover two weeks' worth of meals
- Use fruit and nuts for snacks

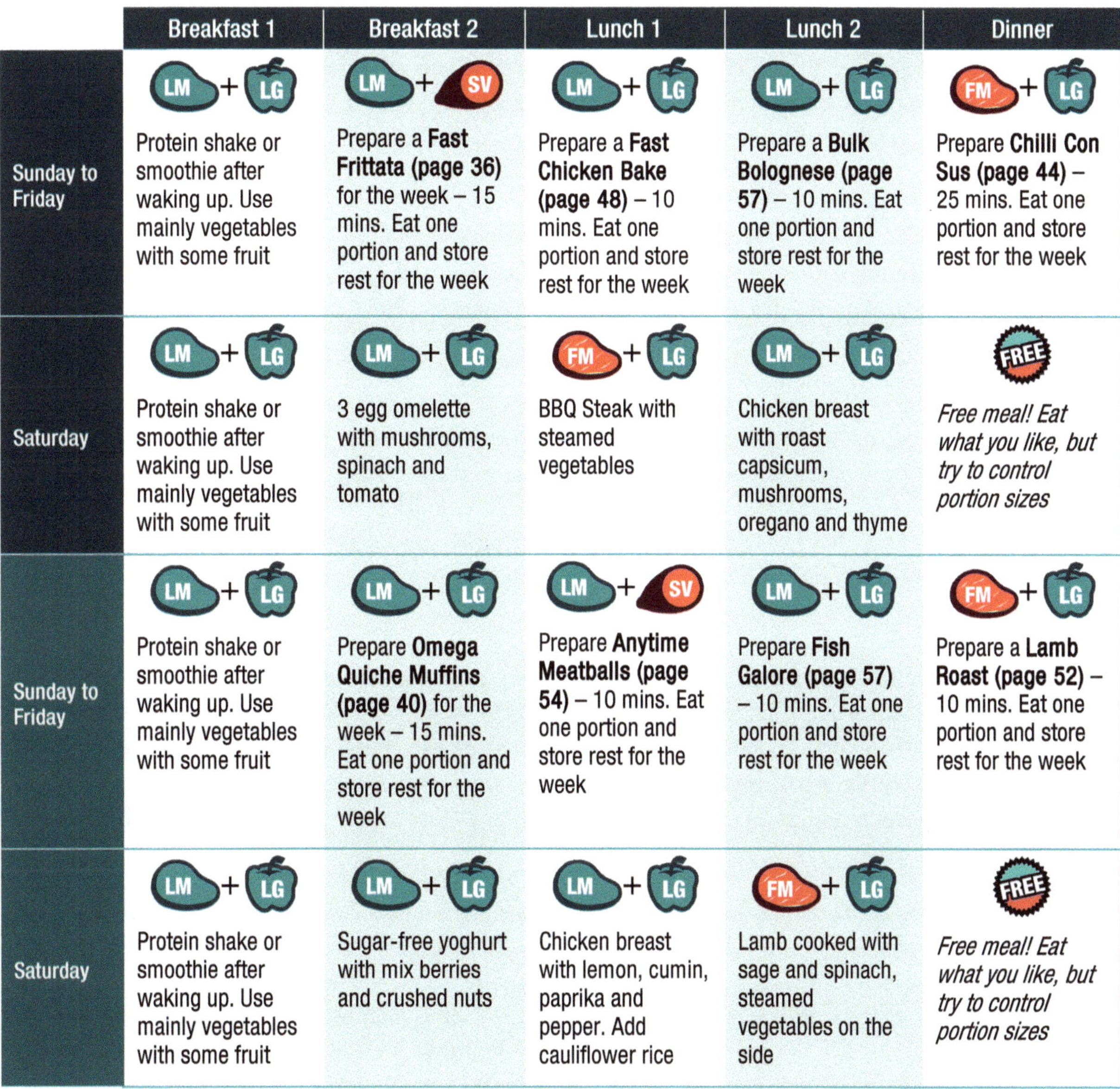

	Breakfast 1	Breakfast 2	Lunch 1	Lunch 2	Dinner
Sunday to Friday	LM + LG Protein shake or smoothie after waking up. Use mainly vegetables with some fruit	LM + SV Prepare a **Fast Frittata (page 36)** for the week – 15 mins. Eat one portion and store rest for the week	LM + LG Prepare a **Fast Chicken Bake (page 48)** – 10 mins. Eat one portion and store rest for the week	LM + LG Prepare a **Bulk Bolognese (page 57)** – 10 mins. Eat one portion and store rest for the week	FM + LG Prepare **Chilli Con Sus (page 44)** – 25 mins. Eat one portion and store rest for the week
Saturday	LM + LG Protein shake or smoothie after waking up. Use mainly vegetables with some fruit	LM + LG 3 egg omelette with mushrooms, spinach and tomato	FM + LG BBQ Steak with steamed vegetables	LM + LG Chicken breast with roast capsicum, mushrooms, oregano and thyme	FREE *Free meal! Eat what you like, but try to control portion sizes*
Sunday to Friday	LM + LG Protein shake or smoothie after waking up. Use mainly vegetables with some fruit	LM + LG Prepare **Omega Quiche Muffins (page 40)** for the week – 15 mins. Eat one portion and store rest for the week	LM + SV Prepare **Anytime Meatballs (page 54)** – 10 mins. Eat one portion and store rest for the week	LM + LG Prepare **Fish Galore (page 57)** – 10 mins. Eat one portion and store rest for the week	FM + LG Prepare a **Lamb Roast (page 52)** – 10 mins. Eat one portion and store rest for the week
Saturday	LM + LG Protein shake or smoothie after waking up. Use mainly vegetables with some fruit	LM + LG Sugar-free yoghurt with mix berries and crushed nuts	LM + LG Chicken breast with lemon, cumin, paprika and pepper. Add cauliflower rice	FM + LG Lamb cooked with sage and spinach, steamed vegetables on the side	FREE *Free meal! Eat what you like, but try to control portion sizes*

2.2 Think Free Pyramid – Insulin optimisation

For many, the thought of giving up sweet serotonin-releasing sugar and grains is just too much to bear. But fear not! There are ways to adapt our diets to incorporate sugar and grains in a healthy way. But there are two caveats about sugar and grains we need to keep in mind:

- They increase serotonin in the brain which motivates you to eat more[9]. This is why it is so easy to overeat these foods – the brain is wired to crave it[10]!
- They spike insulin levels which cause the body to store fat[11]. The body stores most fat when you eat high-GI foods at the same time as fatty foods

Because of this, controlling intake of grains and sugar requires more self-control than the ***Think Lean Pyramid*** does and you need to be careful of the food groups you eat together. Of course, if you already have a fair amount of discipline and can effectively control your portions, then this food pyramid will give you the freedom to include the full spectrum of foods. Because of this, it is called the ***Think Free Pyramid.***

2.2.1 What it works for

This is great as an alternative to Complete ACM as shown in the Goal Body Matrix. Since it contains grains and sugars, it requires discipline to control your portions. However, by ensuring that we eat the right foods together we can actually optimise insulin release to reduce the ability of foods to be converted to body fat. Overall, this plan is great for:

- If you want to lose weight but it is important to you to have the freedom of adding in grains and sugar, and you have the discipline to not overeat on these foods
- If you are working out and want to improve muscle definition
- If you generally have weight under control and simply want to switch to a healthier eating plan

2.2.2 Why it works

Our bodies mainly store energy as body fat when there is an insulin spike in the presence of fatty foods. This is why foods with a lot of high-GI carbohydrates and dietary fats make us gain weight. These foods include chocolate, ice cream, potato chips, burgers, cookies, fries, and most fast foods. It's the *combination* that we have to avoid, which is why the ***Think Free Pyramid*** is structured in a way that encourages you to eat the right foods together so that you can lose weight more efficiently. There are two parts that make it work:

- **Stick to high-fibre, wholegrain foods.** Many products say "wholegrain" on the package, but really mean that the product *contains* wholegrains along with a whole bunch of other unhealthy stuff. A prime example is bread which often contains some wholegrains to make it look healthy, while the rest is still a refined wheat product that is bad for your health. You want real wholegrain foods – not the pretend stuff! This might take a bit of searching around with breads, but easier foods include oats and brown rice as great choices.
- **Eat grain products and sugar together with low fat foods.** Sugar and grains are usually higher on the glycaemic index and thus cause an insulin spike. The insulin spike on its own doesn't cause body fat storage, but does store body fat when dietary fats are being digested as well. This

means something like bread with olive oil is the perfect mixture to store body fat. It is much better to eat high-GI products like bread with low fat foods like chicken breast and other lean meats.

The combination of these two factors means you can still include grain products with a bit of sugar without having to worry about adding body fat. Keep in mind that the combination of high-GI carbohydrates and dietary fats is the most desirable taste to the brain (good examples are chocolate, donuts and ice cream), so you'll need to be a bit more conscious about portion sizes when it comes to grains.

This is a great way to ease into healthy eating and can be a permanent plan for weight management. If you want to achieve lower body fat or find this doesn't work for you to lose weight, try the ***Think Lean Pyramid*** instead. It all comes down to your goals and what you want to achieve – remember to eat towards your goals!

2.2.3 Guidelines

As before, the size of the segments in the pyramid below indicate the relative number of calories you get from each food group. We want loads of vegetables still for their health boosting effect, along with protein with every meal to keep us full and metabolism going strong.

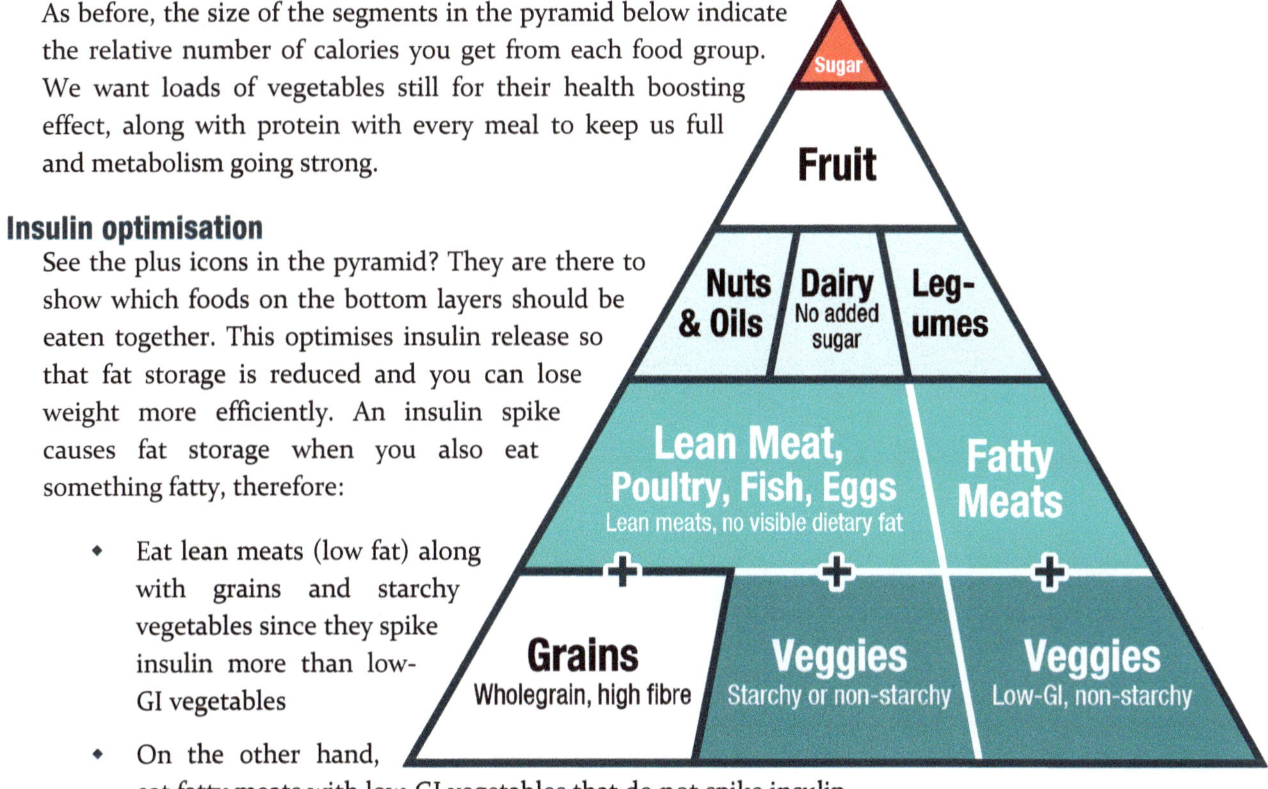

Insulin optimisation

See the plus icons in the pyramid? They are there to show which foods on the bottom layers should be eaten together. This optimises insulin release so that fat storage is reduced and you can lose weight more efficiently. An insulin spike causes fat storage when you also eat something fatty, therefore:

- Eat lean meats (low fat) along with grains and starchy vegetables since they spike insulin more than low-GI vegetables
- On the other hand, eat fatty meats with low-GI vegetables that do not spike insulin

Use this approach with your main meals through the day and keep that same concept in mind with other fatty foods to optimise insulin spikes.

When it comes to losing weight and weight maintenance, the total calories should come in around 1300 to 1700 depending on how much you eat. If you stick to the portion guidelines below you shouldn't have to count calories, but you'll need to be disciplined. If you don't want to worry about being disciplined, then the Automatic Calorie Management aspect of the ***Think Lean Pyramid*** might be more your thing. However, if you can stay in control with your eating, this food pyramid will allow you to eat all types of foods.

Think Free Pyramid - Main food groups

Use the table below for a general indication on how much to eat with each meal. As before, the exact amounts you eat will vary depending on your goal, so use the meal plans further down to work out how much to eat. ***Also, see the end of the book for full food lists for this food pyramid.***

Food type	Portions	Notes
Lean meats & eggs	One or two servings for a meal.	Eat lean meats and eggs with grains and starchy vegetables to optimise your insulin response. LM
Fatty meats	One or two servings for a meal.	Fatty meats have visible strips of dietary fat and can result in body fat storage if you eat it with high-GI foods like grains. Because of that, eat these along with low-GI, non-starchy vegetables. FM
Low-GI vegetables	Three servings for a meal.	Eat as much as you want! The more, the better. LG
Starchy vegetables	Two or three servings.	Eat with lean meats to optimise insulin response. Stick to whole foods and avoid white potatoes. SV
Wholegrains	Two or three servings for a meal.	Eat with lean meats. Wholegrain foods close to their original forms are the best, such as rolled oats (not quick oats), brown rice, quinoa, and so on. If you need more calories, whole wheat pasta or bread can also work, but check your progress so that you don't pick up body fat as well. WG
Nuts	One serving per day.	Use as snacks or to garnish meals.
Oils	Use oils sparingly.	Coconut oil works best as it is low in omega-6. Sunflower and most other plant oils are high in omega-6, so try to limit these. Butter is an alternative for cooking. Extra virgin olive oil is a better choice than other plant oils.
Dairy	One serving per day.	Unsweetened dairy products are a good addition as they are the primary source of calcium in our diets. If you can't tolerate dairy, consider taking a Calcium supplement.
Legumes	One serving per day.	Use as an addition to a meal, or to replace grains or starchy vegetables.
Fruit	One serving or one piece of fruit a day.	While other foods are generally healthier and more nutritious than fruit, fruit is always preferable to sweets and high-GI grain foods!

Think Free Pyramid - Other foods

Think Free includes wholegrain foods and a bit of sugar, allowing you to eat from all food groups. Of course the key is to have control and stick to your goal, so you need more self-discipline to stick to this food pyramid. The table below shows other food groups you might be considering, with the good ones in green, and those to limit in grey. 'Limit' foods can also be eaten as part of the weekly free meal, though try to keep the free meal to a reasonable size.

Food type	Include?	Notes
Water	Yes	Make this your drink of choice! Drink more to help you feel full.
Herbs & spices	Yes	Eat as much as you like! This is a great way to spice up foods in a guilt-free way.
Sweeteners	Yes	Try a natural sweetener like xylitol, stevia or erythritol. Chewing gum and sweets that use sweeteners are fine.
Caffeine	Limit	Stick to one cup of coffee per day, preferably at the start of the day.
Alcohol	Limit	White wines and champagne are often better choices. Cut out cocktails and mixers as they are high in sugars. Try to keep to just one or two glasses a week.
Sugar, sweets, soft drinks, etc.	Limit	Limit sugar to around 1.5 teaspoons (7g) in a day.
Chocolate	Limit	Limit chocolates for better results. Because they contain both sugar and dietary fat, they quickly cause body fat storage. Sugar free chocolate is something you can enjoy more regularly.

2.2.4 Meal plan templates

The meal plan templates below show you what kind of foods to eat at each meal, depending on the number of meals you need per day to reach your goal. Each meal shows you what kind of foods to have, giving you a template to build other meal plans around. Of course it also includes suggestions of recipes to eat so you can get started straight away.

*Think Free: **3-Meal Plan Template***

- Do your meal prep on Sundays. Eat one portion and save the rest for the week days
- On Saturdays you can have other meals, though stick to eating the right food groups for two of the three meals at least
- For **variety**, try cooking more recipes on Sunday so that you can eat different meals through the week. Otherwise you can skip the dinner meal prep and make something different each night
- Use fruit and nuts for snacks

	Breakfast	Lunch	Dinner
Sunday to Friday	LM + SV Prepare a **Fast Frittata (page 36)** for the week – 15 mins. Eat one portion and store rest for the week	FM + LG Prepare a **Fast Chicken Bake (page 48)** – 10 mins. Eat one portion and store rest for the week	LM + WG Prepare **Chilli Con Sus (page 44)** – 25 mins. Eat one portion and store rest for the week
Saturday	LM + WG 3 egg omelette with mushrooms, spinach and tomato on whole wheat toast	FM + LG BBQ Steak with steamed vegetables	FREE *Free meal! Eat what you like, but try to control portion sizes*
Sunday to Friday	FM + LG Prepare **Omega Quiche Muffins (page 40)** for the week – 15 mins. Eat one portion and store rest for the week	LM + WG Prepare **Anytime Meatballs (page 54)** – 10 mins. Eat one portion and store rest for the week	LM + SV Prepare a **Lamb Roast (page 52)** – 10 mins. Eat one portion and store rest for the week
Saturday	LM + WG 2 eggs on rye toast with avocado & cracked pepper	FM + LG Grilled lamb with steamed vegetables	FREE *Free meal! Eat what you like, but try to control portion sizes*
Sunday to Friday	FM + LG Prepare **Poached Chicken Salad (page 56)** for the week – 15 mins. Eat one portion and store rest for the week	LM + SV Prepare **Turkey Burgers (page 46)** – 20 mins. Eat one portion and store rest for the week	LM + WG Prepare a **Beef Stew (page 50)** – 25 mins. Eat one portion and store rest for the week
Saturday	FM + LG 3 scrambled eggs with 2 strips of bacon with sautéed mushrooms and tomato	LM + WG Chicken breast with lemon, cumin, paprika and pepper with brown rice	FREE *Free meal! Eat what you like, but try to control portion sizes*

Think Free: ***4-Meal Plan Template***

- Do your meal prep on Sundays. Eat one portion and save the rest for the week days
- On Saturdays you can have other meals, though stick to eating the right food groups for three of the four meals at least
- Use fruit and nuts for snacks
- **Speed it up** by replacing Lunch 1 or Lunch 2 with a protein shake or smoothie

	Breakfast	Lunch 1	Lunch 2	Dinner
Sunday to Friday	LM + SV Prepare a **Fast Frittata (page 36)** for the week – 15 mins. Eat one portion and store rest for the week	FM + LG Prepare a **Fast Chicken Bake (page 48)** – 10 mins. Eat one portion and store rest for the week	LM + LG Prepare a **Bulk Bolognese (page 57)** – 10 mins. Eat one portion and store rest for the week	LM + WG Prepare **Chilli Con Sus (page 44)** – 25 mins. Eat one portion and store rest for the week
Saturday	LM + WG 3 egg omelette with mushrooms, spinach and tomato on whole wheat toast	FM + LG BBQ Steak with steamed vegetables	LM + LG Chicken breast with roast capsicum, mushrooms, oregano and rosemary	FREE *Free meal! Eat what you like, but try to control portion sizes*
Sunday to Friday	FM + LG Prepare **Omega Quiche Muffins (page 40)** for the week – 15 mins. Eat one portion and store rest for the week	LM + WG Prepare **Anytime Meatballs (page 54)** – 10 mins. Eat one portion and store rest for the week	LM + LG Prepare **Fish Galore (page 57)** – 10 mins. Eat one portion and store rest for the week	LM + SV Prepare a **Lamb Roast (page 52)** – 10 mins. Eat one portion and store rest for the week
Saturday	LM + WG 2 eggs on rye toast with avocado and cracked pepper	LM + LG Grilled salmon with steamed vegetables	FM + LG Lamb cooked with sage and spinach, steamed vegetables on the side	FREE *Free meal! Eat what you like, but try to control portion sizes*
Sunday to Friday	FM + LG Prepare **Poached Chicken Salad (page 56)** for the week – 15 mins. Eat one portion and store rest for the week	LM + LG Prepare **Turkey Burgers (page 46)** – 20 mins. Eat one portion and store rest for the week	LM + SV Prepare **Fast Chicken Bake (page 48)** – 10 mins. Eat one portion and store rest for the week	LM + WG Prepare a **Beef Stew (page 50)** – 25 mins. Eat one portion and store rest for the week
Saturday	FM + LG 3 scrambled eggs with 2 strips of bacon and sautéed mushrooms	LM + WG Chicken breast with lemon, cumin, paprika, pepper and brown rice	LM + LG Grilled salmon with steamed vegetables	FREE *Free meal! Eat what you like, but try to control portion sizes*

Think Free: ***5-Meal Plan Template***

- Do your meal prep on Sundays. Eat one portion and save the rest for the week days
- On Saturdays you can have other meals, though stick to eating the right food groups for four of the five meals at least
- For **variety**, try cooking more recipes on Sunday so that you can eat different meals through the week. Otherwise you can skip the dinner meal prep and make something different each night
- To **speed things up**, try making a double amount of each recipe so you can cover two weeks' worth of meals
- Use fruit and nuts for snacks

	Breakfast 1	Breakfast 2	Lunch 1	Lunch 2	Dinner
Sunday to Friday	LM + LG Protein shake or smoothie after waking up. Use mainly vegetables with some fruit	LM + SV Prepare a **Fast Frittata (page 36)** for the week – 15 mins. Eat one portion and store rest for the week	FM + LG Prepare a **Fast Chicken Bake (page 48)** – 10 mins. Eat one portion and store rest for the week	LM + LG Prepare a **Bulk Bolognese (page 57)** – 10 mins. Eat one portion and store rest for the week	LM + WG Prepare **Chilli Con Sus (page 44)** – 25 mins. Eat one portion and store rest for the week
Saturday	LM + LG Protein shake or smoothie after waking up. Use mainly vegetables with some fruit	LM + WG 3 egg omelette with mushrooms, spinach and tomato on whole wheat toast	FM + LG BBQ Steak with steamed vegetables	LM + LG Chicken breast with roast capsicum, mushrooms, oregano and thyme	FREE *Free meal! Eat what you like, but try to control portion sizes*
Sunday to Friday	LM + LG Protein shake or smoothie after waking up. Use mainly vegetables with some fruit	FM + LG Prepare **Omega Quiche Muffins (page 40)** for the week – 15 mins. Eat one portion and store rest for the week	LM + WG Prepare **Anytime Meatballs (page 54)** – 10 mins. Eat one portion and store rest for the week	LM + LG Prepare **Fish Galore (page 57)** – 10 mins. Eat one portion and store rest for the week	LM + SV Prepare a **Lamb Roast (page 52)** – 10 mins. Eat one portion and store rest for the week
Saturday	LM + LG Protein shake or smoothie after waking up. Use mainly vegetables with some fruit	LM + WG 2 eggs on rye toast with avocado and cracked pepper	LM + LG Grilled salmon with steamed vegetables	FM + LG Lamb cooked with sage and spinach, steamed vegetables on the side	FREE *Free meal! Eat what you like, but try to control portion sizes*

2.3 Think Big Pyramid – Intermittent Carbohydrate Fasting

When it comes to building a more muscular body, or if you naturally have a hard time putting on weight, you need a different type of nutrition. While ACM helps to keep cravings low and naturally reduce how many calories you take in, you need something almost the total opposite if you really want to add muscle mass. So if you're a guy or gal looking to build muscle, this is the food pyramid for you. Designed with much higher carbohydrate content, it powers your body while you build muscle!

2.3.1 What it works for

This section is really for two kinds of people:

- People who want to build muscle and get an athletic body
- People who have a hard time putting on weight overall

Males in particular might have to do this to build muscle faster, and this is especially useful for females who have a hard time putting on weight. And yes, there absolutely are people who struggle to put on weight! For them it can be just has hard to put on weight as it is for other people to lose weight!

The key is to build muscle without adding body fat, which is to many the holy grail of body building. We'll use some new research to achieve this – it can be done!

2.3.2 Why it works

Carbohydrates and protein make a great combination to build muscle, but loads of carbohydrate can lead to unwanted body fat storage. Lucky for us there is tons of data and scientific research showing us a new way! Through research and experimentation, I've developed Intermittent Carbohydrate Fasting (ICF) to build muscle while staying lean.

The concept of ICF is a simple dietary adjustment between workout days and rest days as follows:

- **Workout days** – take in high calories with a high carbohydrate content
- **Rest days** – drop the calories by lowering carbohydrates

Simple enough, but I'm sure you are wondering about the origins of ICF.

I've tried high-carbohydrate diets to build muscle and they definitely work well. The problem, however, is that they have a tendency to add a lot of body fat in the process. My waist size ballooned at a rate faster than my chest, which was definitely not what I was after! On top of that, I had an omega-6 overdose from all the grain foods. All the omega-6 caused systemic inflammation which resulted in me getting sick, frequent headaches and bad asthma... overall not good.

While doing some research, I noticed more and more studies on fasting, including the benefits of intermittent fasting. Separately, I also read that many top bodybuilders were having success on 'carb cycling', which is the idea to eat a lot of carbohydrates on workout days and replace them with dietary fat on rest days. While scientific evidence of carbohydrate cycling is just emerging, I thought there might be some value in the idea, especially if it could give me a way to build muscle without getting a grain overdose along the way!

2.3.2.1 The evidence

Summarising what I found, here are the key points from the research:

- **Study:** A combination of higher carbohydrate and protein intake leads to better protein synthesis for muscle growth[12,13]. This is a long-established principle for building muscle. The increased energy from carbohydrates prevents the body from breaking down proteins for energy, meaning more protein is available for muscle growth
- **Study:** Intermittent fasting through high calorie days and low calorie days has an advantage for weight loss and insulin resistance[14]. While overall caloric restriction is very similar in effectiveness for fat loss, we can take advantage of our need for higher carbohydrate intake for workout days to build muscle
- **Study:** Lower carbohydrate intake during weight loss leads to improved body fat loss while retaining muscle mass[15]. This is how we keep gains but still cut body fat during rest days
- **Study:** Losing body fat fast is best achieved through diets higher in protein[16], thus high protein / low carbohydrate diets are more useful during rest days to quickly cut body fat before the next workout day

Using these inputs, I developed ICF as a way to use the efficiency of intermittent fasting for high-carbohydrate, high-energy workout days to build muscle, while cutting body fat without losing gains on rest days. This also helps to balance omega-3 and omega-6 to control systemic inflammation (explained in detail in Think Lean Method) since grain foods tend to have much more omega-6 that causes inflammation, while the rest day meals help to restore balance. There is still a lot of research that needs to be done on intermittent fasting, but in the meantime we can use these principles to get results. Personally, ICF has helped me to build muscle without adding body fat, so try it and see for yourself!

2.3.2.2 Applying ICF

To use ICF we actually need two eating plans – one for workout days, and one for rest days. We can use the Think Lean food pyramid as described earlier, and supplement that with a new Think Big food pyramid for workout days. So roughly you'll have an eating plan as follows:

- **Workout days**, around four days a week – Think Big food pyramid
- **Rest days**, for the other three days a week – Think Lean food pyramid

The Think Big pyramid has loads of carbohydrates in it to fuel workouts and muscle growth, while the Think Lean pyramid is high in protein and lower in carbohydrates to keep muscle gains while cutting body fat. Due to the natural caloric restrictive nature of the Think Lean pyramid, you might be dropping about 1000 calories on rest days. So if workout days are around 2500 calories for example, rest days would be about 1500. To make this easy without having to count calories, simply follow the meal plans included below.

If you are looking to build a lot of muscle fast and aren't worried about adding body fat, then you can simply do the Think Big food pyramid all week long. You might also have to eat around six meals a day and have to start counting calories to optimise your results, along with spending much more time in the gym. This is much more time consuming, and again I'd advise to work with a trainer if you'd like to take this approach. Generally I would not recommend this approach for overall health, and personally I favour faster and more efficient meals and workouts, so stick to the guidelines below if you want to save time and still get great results!

2.3.3 Guidelines

The Think Big food pyramid is mainly focused on getting the right macronutrients (carbohydrates, protein and dietary fats) to fuel highly effective workouts. This means eating lots of carbohydrates so that you don't run out of energy. When you are on this plan, you may need to eat more frequently to get enough nutrients. This may be more the case for men, who generally need a higher caloric intake than women. Personally I go for around five meals a day, but you can experiment on yourself to see what gives you better results.

Again the segment size indicates the relative number of calories to get from each food group. The ratios of the main food groups are a simple rule you can follow to prepare your meals:

- 2.5 parts wholegrain or starchy vegetables
- 2 parts protein
- 1 part low-GI vegetables

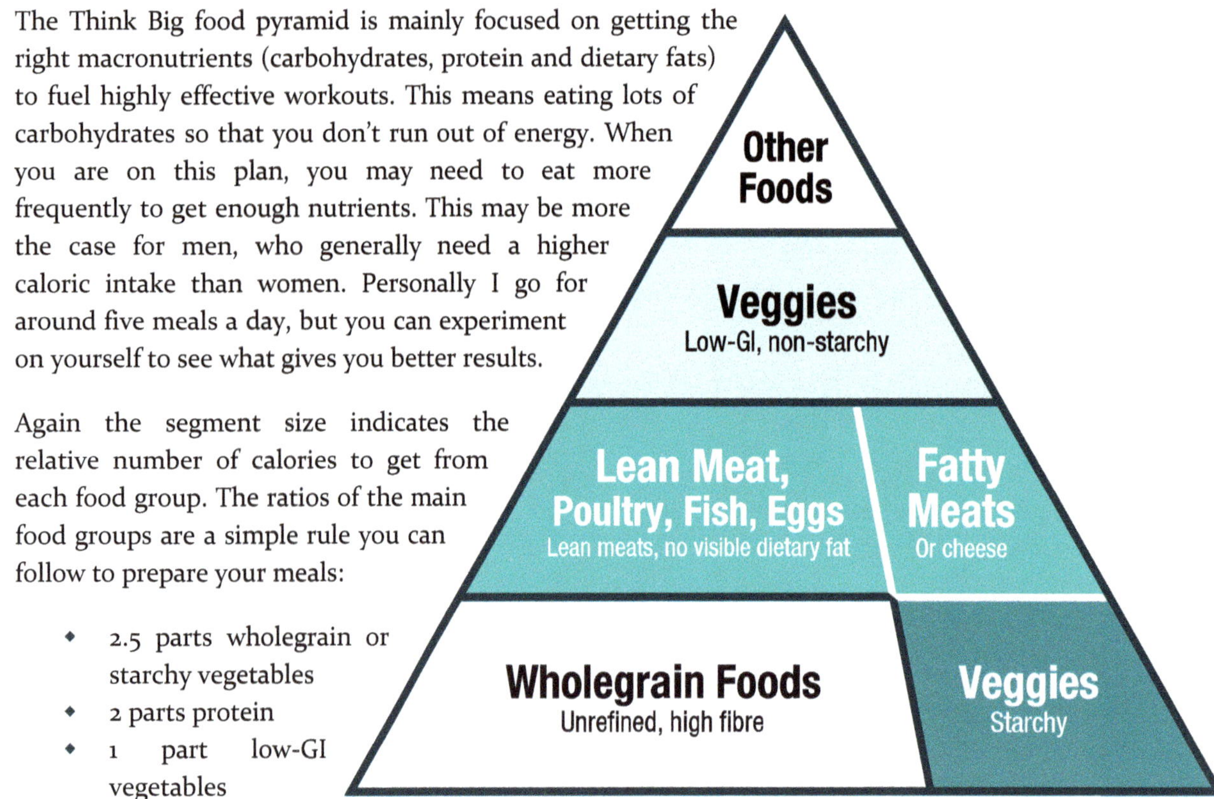

Wholegrain foods, starchy vegetables and protein sources provide your macronutrients and most vitamins and minerals, while the low-GI vegetables fill in the gaps. Below is the guide for the Think Big food pyramid. This is what you will eat on workout days. To put it all together (along with rest day meals) simply follow the meal plans further down.

Think Big Food Pyramid - Main food groups

Adding on more muscle mass means you need to eat bigger meals with more carbohydrates. Because of that, the main difference between this and the other meal plans is that it includes more wholegrain foods so you get the fuel you need to grow. The table below gives a more detailed view of how many servings to have per meal or per day. Use the meal plans for a more precise view of how much to eat. ***Also, see the end of the book for full food lists for this food pyramid.***

Food type	Portions	Notes
Lean meats & eggs	Two servings for a meal.	Eat lean meats, fish and eggs with grains to optimise your insulin response, minimise fat storage and help muscle growth. LM
Fatty meats	Two servings for a meal.	Include as one of every three meals. Avoid eating with grains to better control insulin response. FM
Low-GI vegetables	One serving for a meal.	Eat one serving with each meal for additional micronutrients. LG

Starchy vegetables	Two to three servings.	Eat starchy vegetables along with fatty meats. You can also eat starchy vegetables instead of grain foods. SV
Wholegrains	Two to three servings.	Eat with lean meats. Wholegrain foods still close to its original form are the best, such as rolled oats (not quick oats), brown rice, quinoa, and so on. If you need more calories, whole wheat pasta or bread can also work, but check your progress so that you don't pick up body fat as well. WG
Nuts	Less than one serving per day.	Use as snacks or to garnish meals.
Oils	Use oils sparingly. Max one teaspoon per day.	Coconut oil works best as it is low in omega-6. Sunflower and olive oils are high in omega-6, so try to limit these. Butter is a healthier alternative for cooking.
Dairy	Less than one serving per day.	Unsweetened dairy products are a good addition as they are the primary source of calcium in our diets. If you can't tolerate dairy, consider taking a Calcium supplement.
Legumes	Less than one serving per day.	Can be used as an alternate fuel source instead of starchy vegetables or grains as they are higher in carbohydrates. They tend to be higher on the Glycaemic Index, so try to eat more other food sources.
Fruit	One serving or one piece of fruit a day.	Fruits are fine to have as a healthy snack during the day!

Think Big Food Pyramid - Other foods

The goal is to build muscle while adding as little body fat as possible, and ideally, to lose body fat while adding muscle mass. This gives you an awesomely defined look. To achieve this, we need to cut back on sugars and snacks like chocolates, biscuits, etc. Use the table below to see where these kinds of foods fit in. Good foods are in green, foods to limit in grey, and foods to avoid in red. As always, you can still include all these foods in a free meal each week, but try to keep it to a reasonable size.

Food type	Notes
Water	Make this your drink of choice! Drink more to help you feel full.
Herbs & spices	Eat as much as you like! This is a great way to spice up foods in a guilt-free way.
Sweeteners	Generally try to cut out sweet foods, but if you really want something sweet, try a natural sweetener like xylitol, stevia or erythritol. Chewing gum and sweets that use sweeteners are fine.
Caffeine	Stick to one cup of coffee per day, preferably at the start of the day.
Alcohol	White wines and champagne are often better choices. Cut out cocktails and mixers as they are high in sugars. Try to keep to just one or two glasses a week.
Sugar, sweets, soft drinks, etc.	Go sugar free! Cut out any foods with added sugar.
Chocolate	Most contain sugar and are highly processed, so limit these to free meals. Sugar free chocolate is something you can enjoy more regularly.

2.3.4 Meal plan templates

To implement ICF, you will switch between the Think Big Pyramid for workout days and the Think Lean Pyramid for rest days. So to reflect this, the meal plan templates will swap between them to show you how to do this simply and efficiently. As before, these are set up as templates, allowing you to design your own plans using the adjustable recipes included.

Think BIG ICF: **4-Meal Plan Template**

- Do your meal prep on Sundays. Eat one portion and save the rest for the week days
- On Saturdays you can have other meals, though stick to eating the right food groups for three of the four meals at least
- Use fruit and nuts for snacks
- To **speed things up**, try making a double amount of each recipe so you can cover two weeks' worth of meals
- You can also replace Lunch 1 or Lunch 2 with a protein shake or smoothie
- ***Remember to eat grains only on workout days***

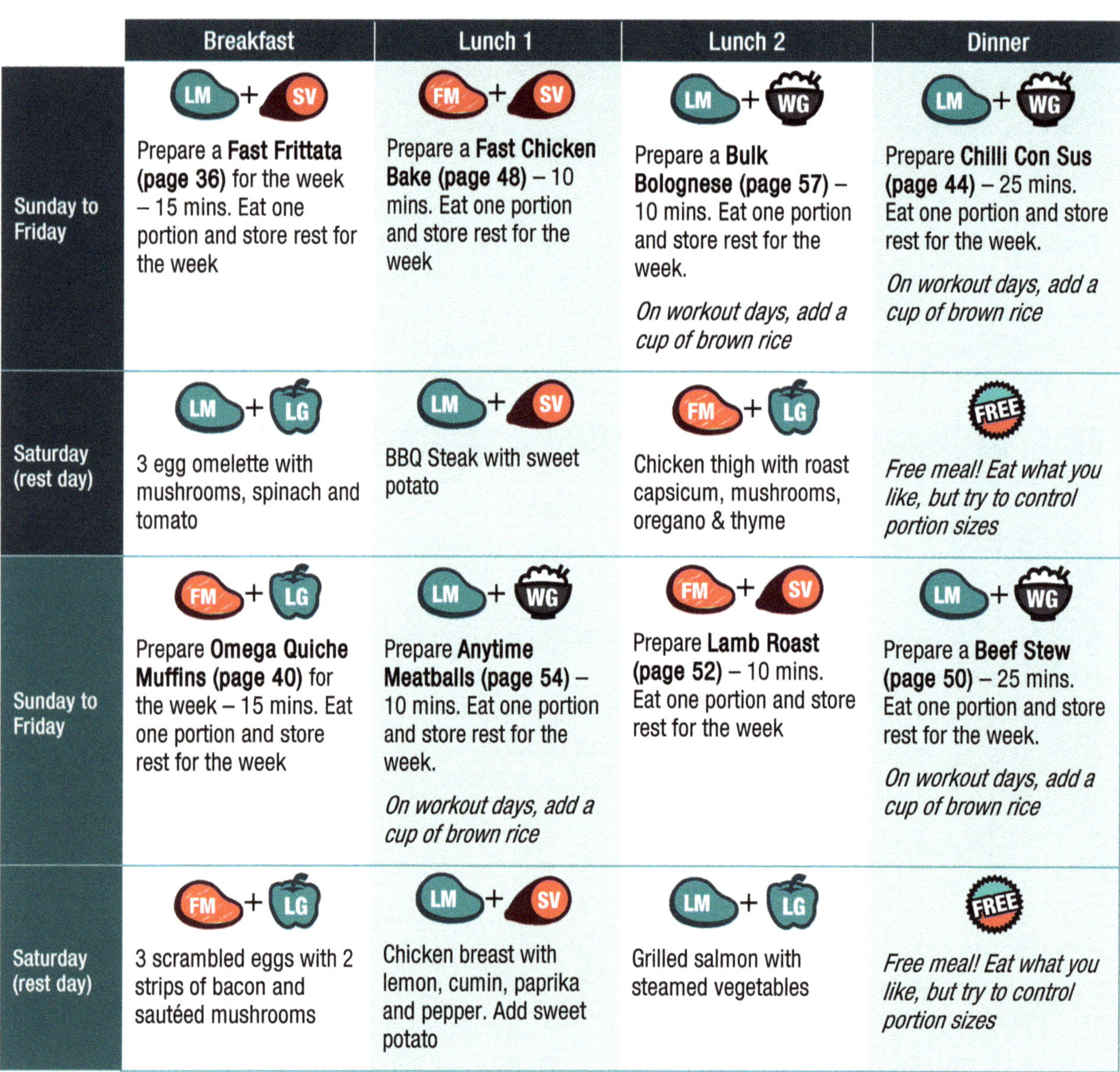

	Breakfast	Lunch 1	Lunch 2	Dinner
Sunday to Friday	LM + SV Prepare a **Fast Frittata (page 36)** for the week – 15 mins. Eat one portion and store rest for the week	FM + SV Prepare a **Fast Chicken Bake (page 48)** – 10 mins. Eat one portion and store rest for the week	LM + WG Prepare a **Bulk Bolognese (page 57)** – 10 mins. Eat one portion and store rest for the week. *On workout days, add a cup of brown rice*	LM + WG Prepare **Chilli Con Sus (page 44)** – 25 mins. Eat one portion and store rest for the week. *On workout days, add a cup of brown rice*
Saturday (rest day)	LM + LG 3 egg omelette with mushrooms, spinach and tomato	LM + SV BBQ Steak with sweet potato	FM + LG Chicken thigh with roast capsicum, mushrooms, oregano & thyme	FREE *Free meal! Eat what you like, but try to control portion sizes*
Sunday to Friday	FM + LG Prepare **Omega Quiche Muffins (page 40)** for the week – 15 mins. Eat one portion and store rest for the week	LM + WG Prepare **Anytime Meatballs (page 54)** – 10 mins. Eat one portion and store rest for the week. *On workout days, add a cup of brown rice*	FM + SV Prepare **Lamb Roast (page 52)** – 10 mins. Eat one portion and store rest for the week	LM + WG Prepare a **Beef Stew (page 50)** – 25 mins. Eat one portion and store rest for the week. *On workout days, add a cup of brown rice*
Saturday (rest day)	FM + LG 3 scrambled eggs with 2 strips of bacon and sautéed mushrooms	LM + SV Chicken breast with lemon, cumin, paprika and pepper. Add sweet potato	LM + LG Grilled salmon with steamed vegetables	FREE *Free meal! Eat what you like, but try to control portion sizes*

Think BIG ICF: ***5-Meal Plan Template***

- Do your meal prep on Sundays. Eat one portion and save the rest for the week days
- On Saturdays you can have other meals, though stick to eating the right food groups for four of the five meals at least
- Use fruit and nuts for snacks
- To **speed things up**, try making a double amount of each recipe so you can cover two weeks' worth of meals
- You can also replace Lunch 1 or Lunch 2 with a protein shake or smoothie
- ***Remember to eat grains only on workout days***

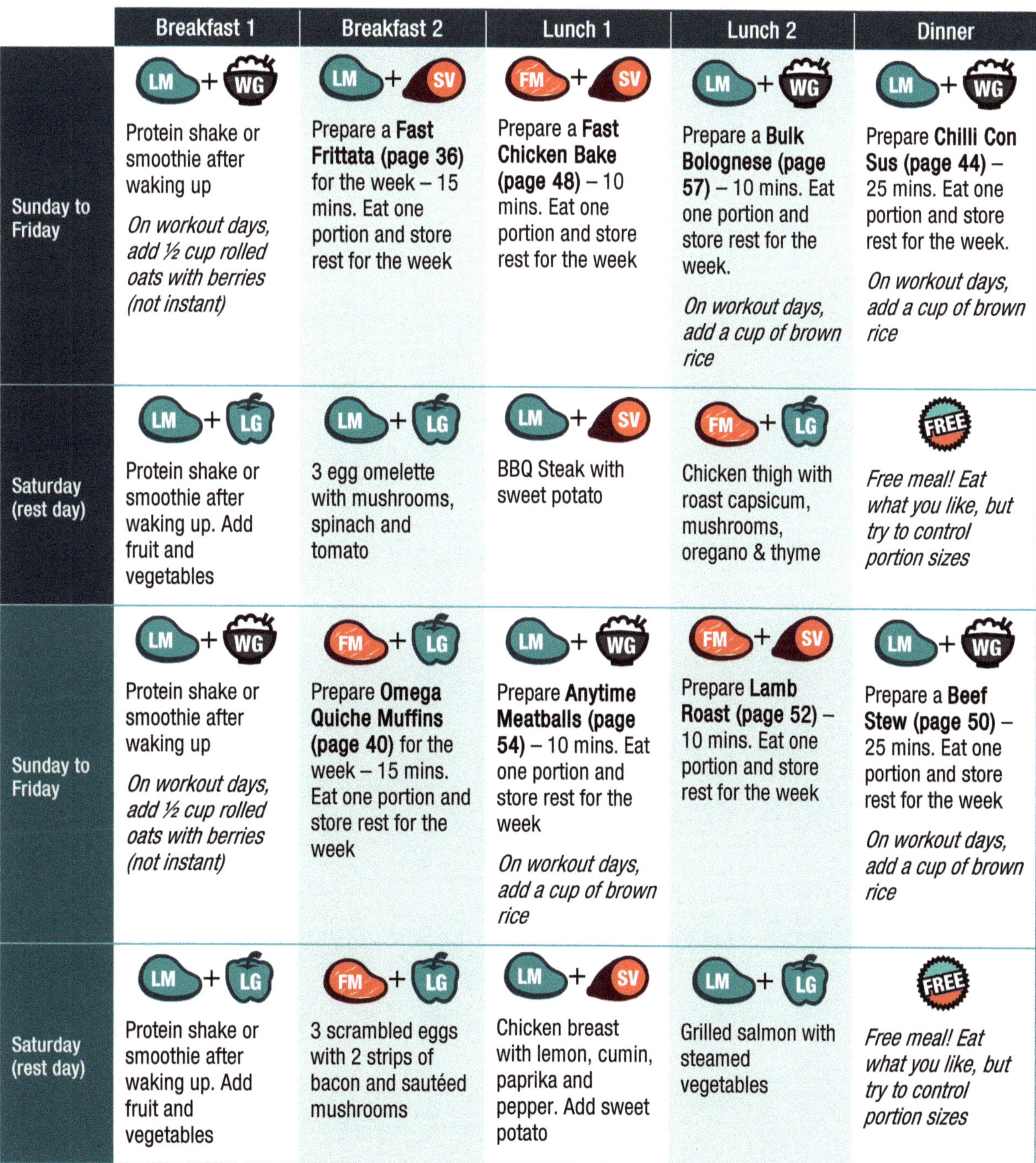

	Breakfast 1	Breakfast 2	Lunch 1	Lunch 2	Dinner
Sunday to Friday	LM + WG Protein shake or smoothie after waking up *On workout days, add ½ cup rolled oats with berries (not instant)*	LM + SV Prepare a **Fast Frittata (page 36)** for the week – 15 mins. Eat one portion and store rest for the week	FM + SV Prepare a **Fast Chicken Bake (page 48)** – 10 mins. Eat one portion and store rest for the week	LM + WG Prepare a **Bulk Bolognese (page 57)** – 10 mins. Eat one portion and store rest for the week. *On workout days, add a cup of brown rice*	LM + WG Prepare **Chilli Con Sus (page 44)** – 25 mins. Eat one portion and store rest for the week. *On workout days, add a cup of brown rice*
Saturday (rest day)	LM + LG Protein shake or smoothie after waking up. Add fruit and vegetables	LM + LG 3 egg omelette with mushrooms, spinach and tomato	LM + SV BBQ Steak with sweet potato	FM + LG Chicken thigh with roast capsicum, mushrooms, oregano & thyme	FREE *Free meal! Eat what you like, but try to control portion sizes*
Sunday to Friday	LM + WG Protein shake or smoothie after waking up *On workout days, add ½ cup rolled oats with berries (not instant)*	FM + LG Prepare **Omega Quiche Muffins (page 40)** for the week – 15 mins. Eat one portion and store rest for the week	LM + WG Prepare **Anytime Meatballs (page 54)** – 10 mins. Eat one portion and store rest for the week *On workout days, add a cup of brown rice*	FM + SV Prepare **Lamb Roast (page 52)** – 10 mins. Eat one portion and store rest for the week	LM + WG Prepare a **Beef Stew (page 50)** – 25 mins. Eat one portion and store rest for the week *On workout days, add a cup of brown rice*
Saturday (rest day)	LM + LG Protein shake or smoothie after waking up. Add fruit and vegetables	FM + LG 3 scrambled eggs with 2 strips of bacon and sautéed mushrooms	LM + SV Chicken breast with lemon, cumin, paprika and pepper. Add sweet potato	LM + LG Grilled salmon with steamed vegetables	FREE *Free meal! Eat what you like, but try to control portion sizes*

3 Bulk Recipe Templates

Saving time while still eating healthy and delicious meals that help you achieve your goals is what it's all about. These recipes are designed for bulk preparation so that you can quickly make one big batch and get on with your life.

In the previous section, the meal plan templates show you how to put together each meal using specific food groups indicated by icons. You can now match up the icons from the meal plan to the icons on the recipe templates to find the right ingredients and instructions. Importantly, these are all **recipe *templates***, meaning they provide the basic guidelines on how to make them, but beyond that you can experiment and change them to suit your tastes and preferences. Overall the recipes are very adaptable with different ingredients you can use, so you can easily change them around to keep it interesting while working towards your goal.

This is all about helping you find a healthy lifestyle that suits your situation and tastes, so get creative and adjust the recipes. Keep in mind that you need to adjust them within the guidelines, so if you are swapping ingredients, swap them for the same type. For example, if the meal plans call for low-GI vegetables, swap them with any other low-GI vegetables and avoid starchy vegetables or grains. Full lists of foods for each food pyramid are included in the back of the book.

We're mainly focused on the big dishes here, so bulk breakfasts and main courses are what you'll find below. If you'd like more healthy recipes, get the original Think Lean Method from Amazon.com or at www.thinkleanmethod.com for loads more options.

Cooking times

Each recipe has estimated times for 'hands-on' work and cooking time, though you will improve on your hands-on work time each time you cook, i.e. getting the ingredients ready faster, becoming more efficient and so on. If you find yourself with a little bit of a break while things are cooking, start doing the dishes or getting your containers ready so that you can get everything done faster. This way you'll spend less time in the kitchen while still eating delicious and healthy meals!

Storing meals

Keeping meals in the freezer will allow you to keep meals for over a week. To avoid having to defrost too often, take out what you want to eat the next day and put it in the fridge. That way it will slowly thaw overnight while still staying fresh.

Try dividing meals into containers or freezer bags when you finish a batch meal. Freezer bags are an inexpensive way to divide meals and reduce washing up later on. You can store them pressed flat so that they defrost faster and fit more easily in the fridge.

Adding variety

An easy way to add variety is to do one big cooking day on a Sunday and make meals for two, three or four weeks. That way you can eat different meals each day and you don't have to cook again for a few weeks. Another way is to only cook breakfast and lunch, while making different meals each evening. Using different kinds of frozen vegetables is also an easy way to get some extra variety in each day without any extra work. You can make the same recipe each week, but try different ingredients or different cooking methods as well. There are loads of ways to add variety – don't be afraid to experiment!

Conversion tables

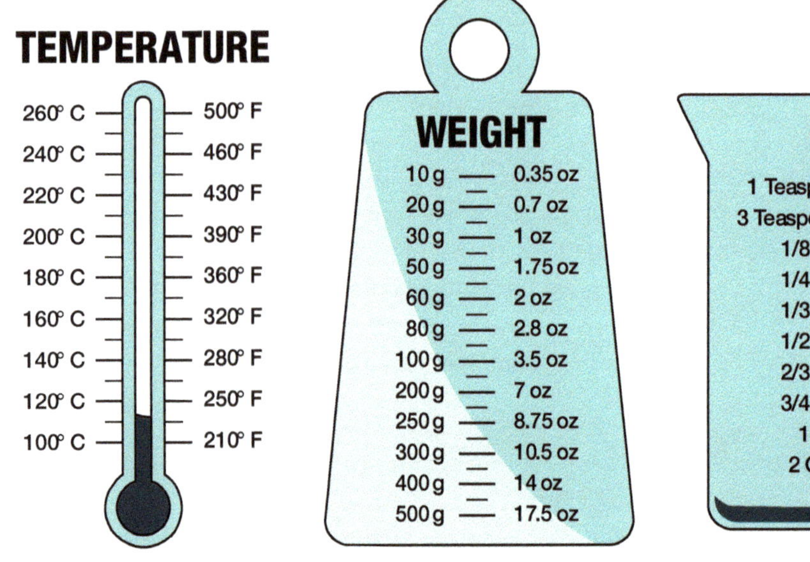

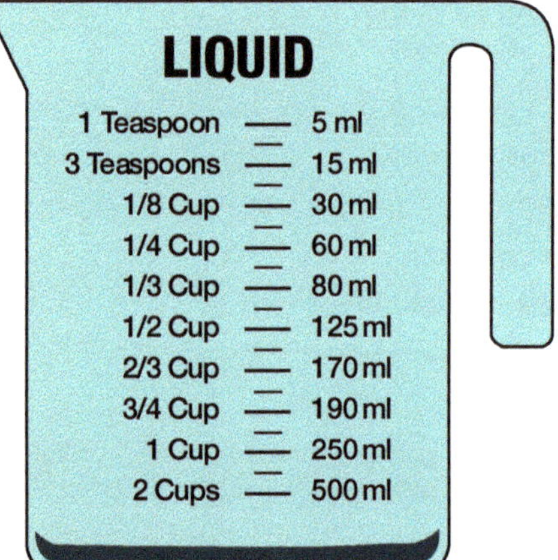
LIQUID
1 Teaspoon — 5 ml
3 Teaspoons — 15 ml
1/8 Cup — 30 ml
1/4 Cup — 60 ml
1/3 Cup — 80 ml
1/2 Cup — 125 ml
2/3 Cup — 170 ml
3/4 Cup — 190 ml
1 Cup — 250 ml
2 Cups — 500 ml

Recipe Templates

Breakfasts

Mains

Other bulk meal ideas

Fast Frittata

Prep time: **15 mins** - Cook time: **35 mins** - Servings: **6**

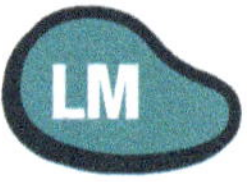

Lean meats

- 24 fresh eggs

OR

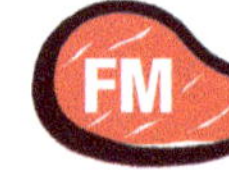

Fatty meats

- 24 fresh eggs
- 100g bacon, fried in butter and diced

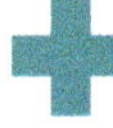

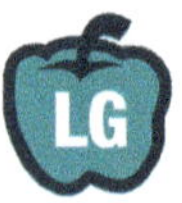

Low-GI veggies

- 3 zucchinis **OR** 5 bunches of broccolini, diced (400g)
- 2 tomatoes, sliced (200g)
- 100g spinach

OR

Starchy veggies

- 1 medium sweet potato, cooked in microwave for 9 minutes on high, diced (400g)
- Roasted capsicum, diced (200g)
- 100g spinach

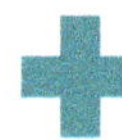

Additional ingredients:

- 250g Mozzarella cheese, grated
- 1 bunch chives **OR** fresh oregano, chopped (30g)
- ½ teaspoon salt
- ½ teaspoon of pepper

Method:

1. Preheat the oven to 150° / 300°F
2. Line a large baking pan with foil, or brush with olive oil
3. Lightly beat the eggs and combine with vegetables in a large baking pan. Stir until mixed
4. Spread cheese evenly on top and garnish with salt, pepper and chives
5. Place in oven and bake for about 35 minutes. Cover with foil after 10 minutes or when golden brown
6. Divide into 6 to 8 servings and store in bags to use during the week

Recipe tips:

- *These do not need to be heated before eating, making them a perfect meal to take anywhere, such as being out at a conference or somewhere without a microwave*
- *You can use an endless combination of vegetables and spices to keep this recipe interesting and fresh. I've eaten this recipe for many weeks in a row by just making small adjustments along the way. It's just so fast and so tasty – hard to beat!*

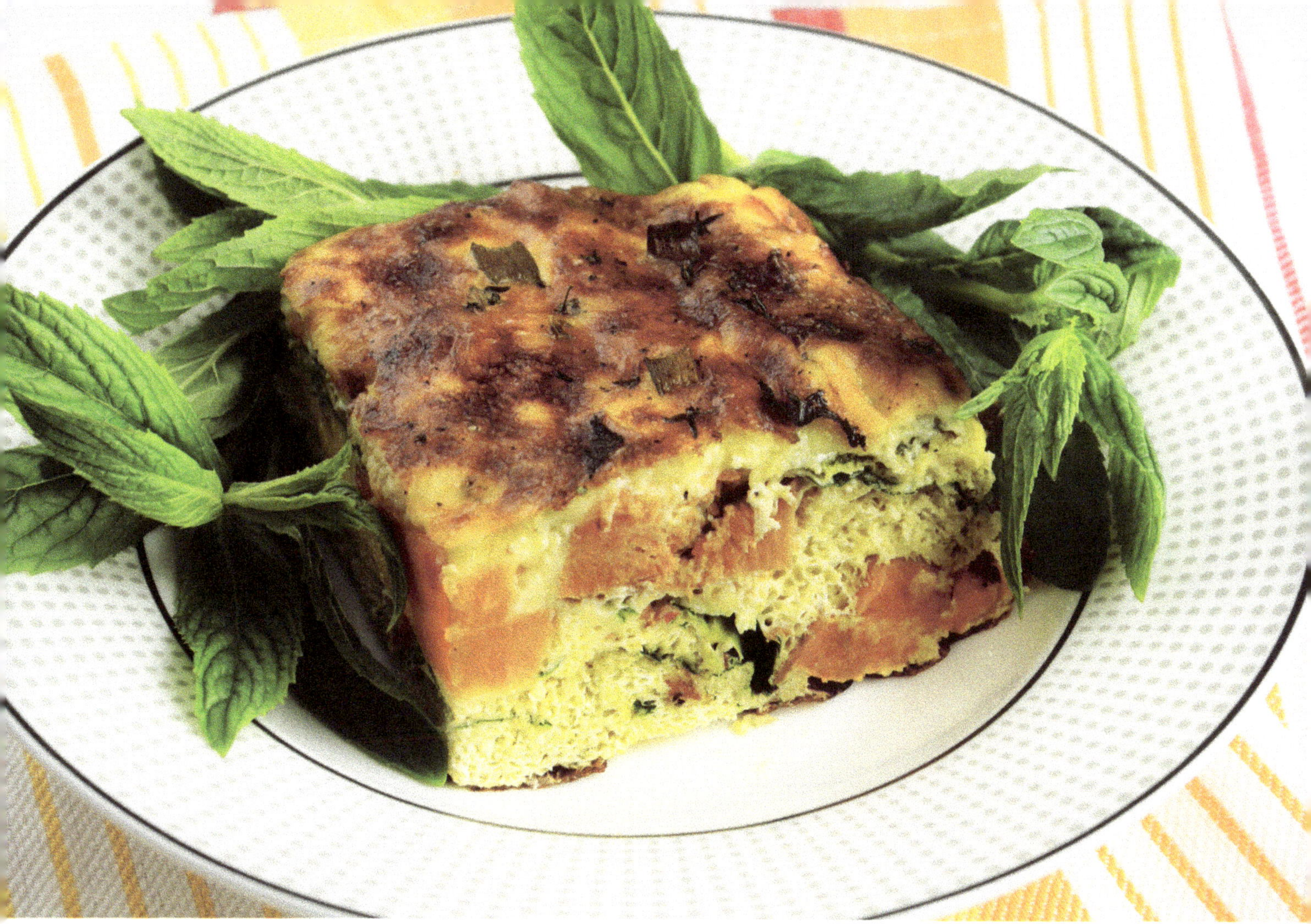

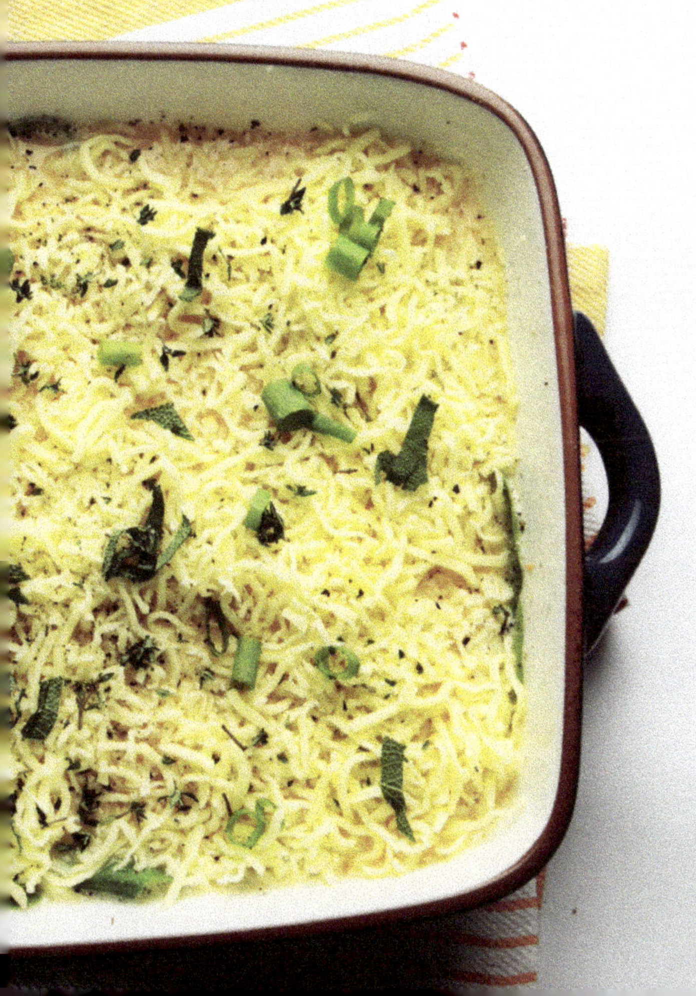
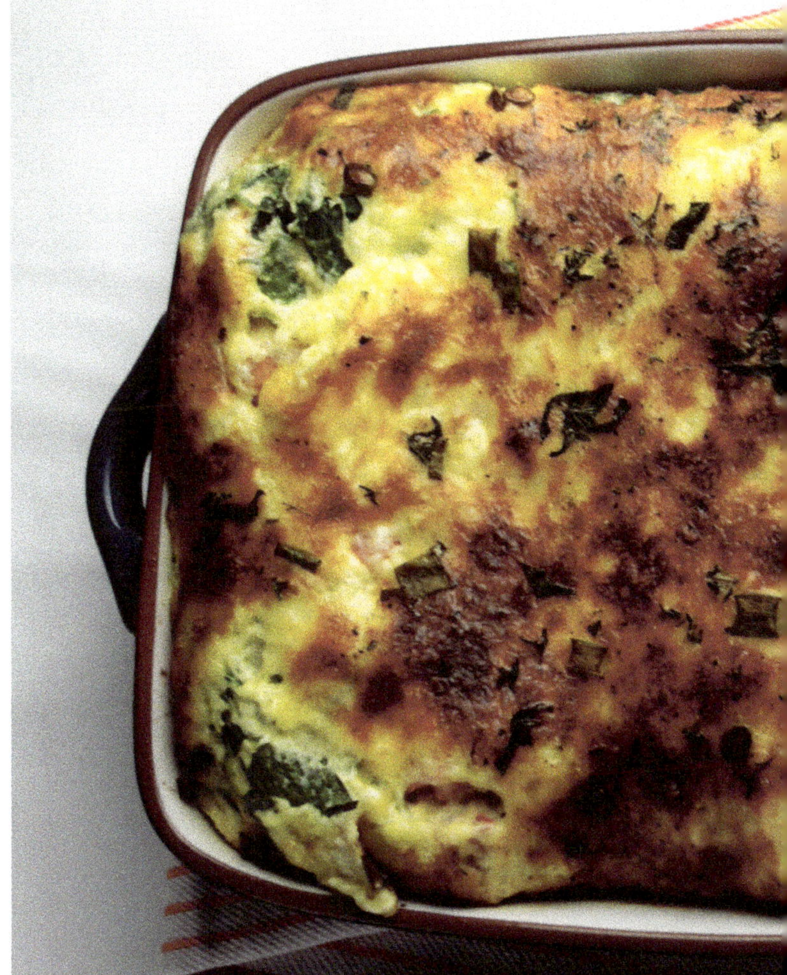

Almond Pancakes

Prep time: **15 mins** - Cook time: **25 mins** - Servings: **5 to 6**

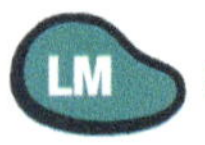

and

- 6 fresh eggs (room temperature)

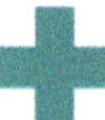

Ingredients:

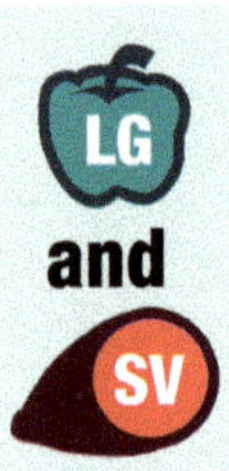

- 3 cups almond flour
- ¾ cup water (sparkling water for extra fluffy pancakes)
- 2 tablespoons melted coconut oil
- 1 teaspoon salt
- 1 teaspoon butter
- 1 teaspoon vanilla extract
- ***Optional:*** *2 punnets of blueberries* ***OR*** *raspberries* ***OR*** *1 large banana, mashed (200g)*

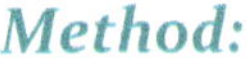

Method:

1. Combine all the ingredients (except the butter) in a mixing bowl and combine with an egg beater. I make these in two batches so the amount is more manageable to pour
2. For extra variation, add blueberries to one batch and mashed banana to the other batch
3. Bring two non-stick pans up to medium heat and pour pancakes that are slightly larger than your spatula (not much larger, otherwise the edges of the pancake might break when flipping)
4. Flip when bubbles form on the uncooked side, or after 3 minutes

Recipe tips:

- *Separate into 5 or 6 servings and store in bags for the week. These can be kept in the freezer for longer periods*
- *These can be eaten cold or warmed in a microwave*
- *Keep in mind that the almond flour contains more dietary fat than usual, so avoid eating these pancakes with any added sugar. That means no honey or maple syrup (unless it is sugar free). Go instead of toppings like sugar free yoghurt, or eat on its own (my choice!)*
- *For a more savoury meal, make the pancakes with a splash of lemon and eat with grated cheese*

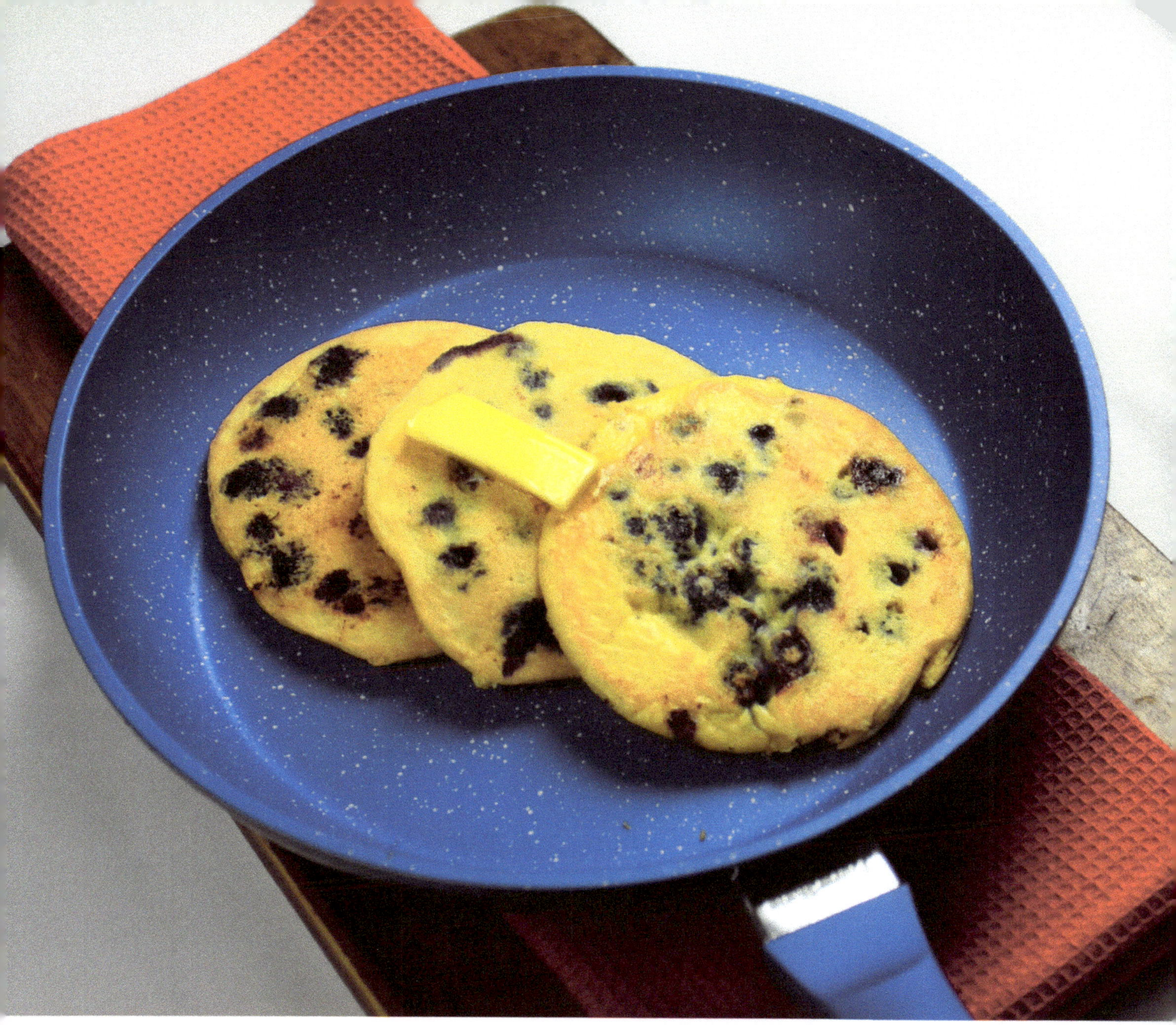

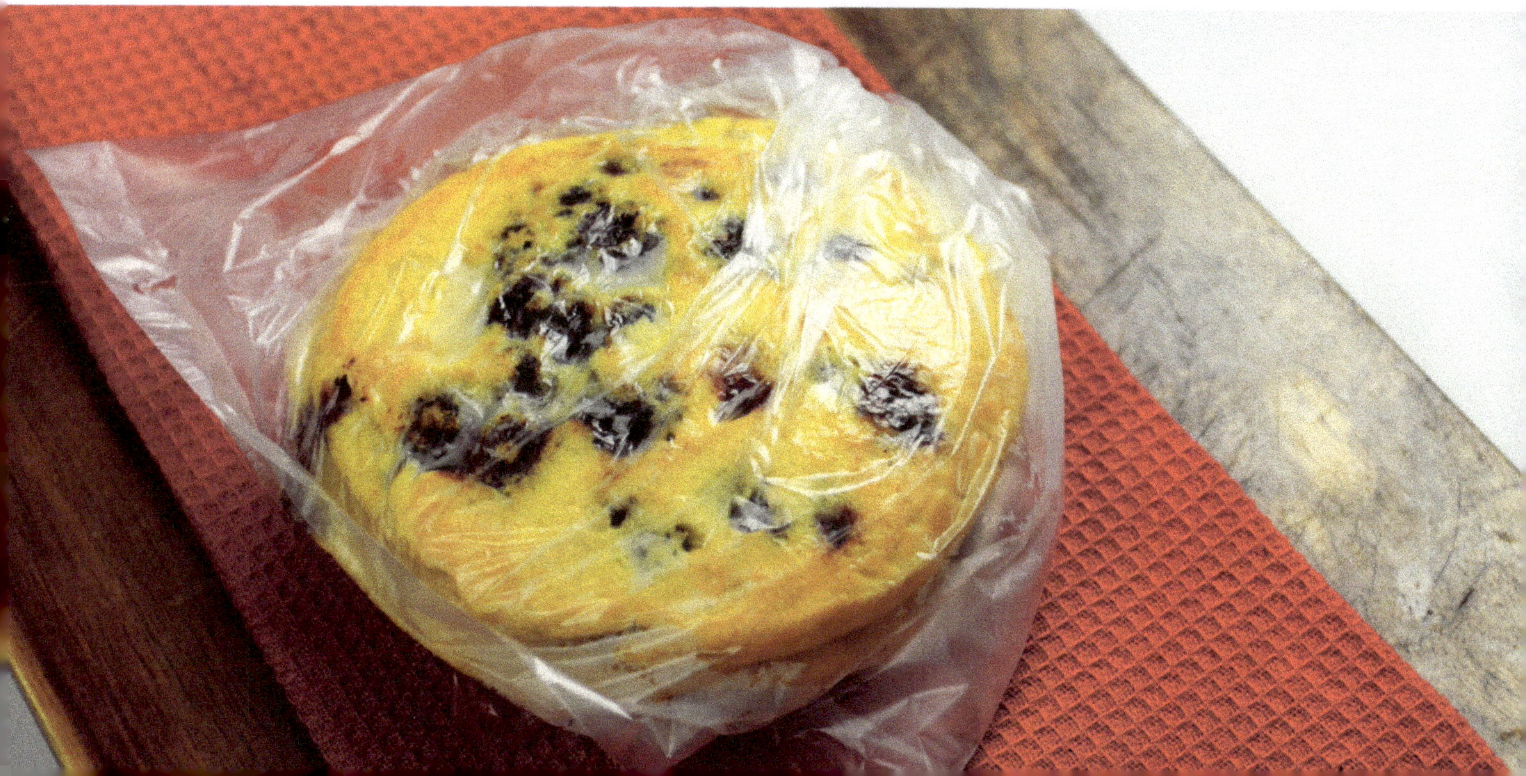

Omega Quiche Muffins

Prep time: **20 mins** - Cook time: **35 mins** - Servings: **6**

Lean meats

- 8 fresh eggs
- 600g smoked salmon **OR** canned salmon **OR** tuna in brine, shredded

OR

Fatty meats

- 8 fresh eggs
- 400g smoked salmon **OR** canned salmon **OR** tuna in brine, shredded
- 200g bacon

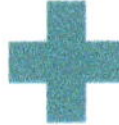

Rest of the ingredients:

- 100g cheddar cheese, grated
- 20g parmesan cheese, grated
- 2 cups coconut cream
- ½ cup coconut flour
- ¼ brown onion, chopped
- 1 teaspoon salt
- Pinch of pepper
- ***Optional:** 3 large capsicums*

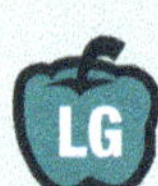

and

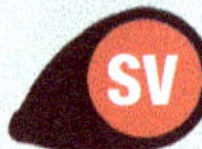

Method:

1. Preheat the oven to 170° / 340°F
2. Lightly beat the eggs in a bowl
3. If making with bacon, fry in a saucepan over medium heat for 5 minutes with onion, let cool slightly and dice
4. Mix the salmon, cheeses, flour, onion (and bacon, if used) and salt in the bowl with eggs and mix until evenly coated
5. Heat the coconut cream on low heat in a saucepan for 2 minutes and mix into the other ingredients
6. Pour mix into a muffin tray. If using capsicums, halve the capsicums, cut out seeds and pour mix into six capsicum halves. Place on a baking tray lined with foil
7. Bake in oven for 30 minutes or until golden brown. Insert a toothpick and check that it comes out clean

Recipe tips:

- *Using a muffin tray is a super simple way to divide meals and ensure fast and even cooking. A flexible tray is easier to use , or line the tray with paper or muffin cups to make them easier to remove*
- *With the muffins, optionally eat a salad made from fresh lettuce, cucumber, tomato and other low-GI vegetables*

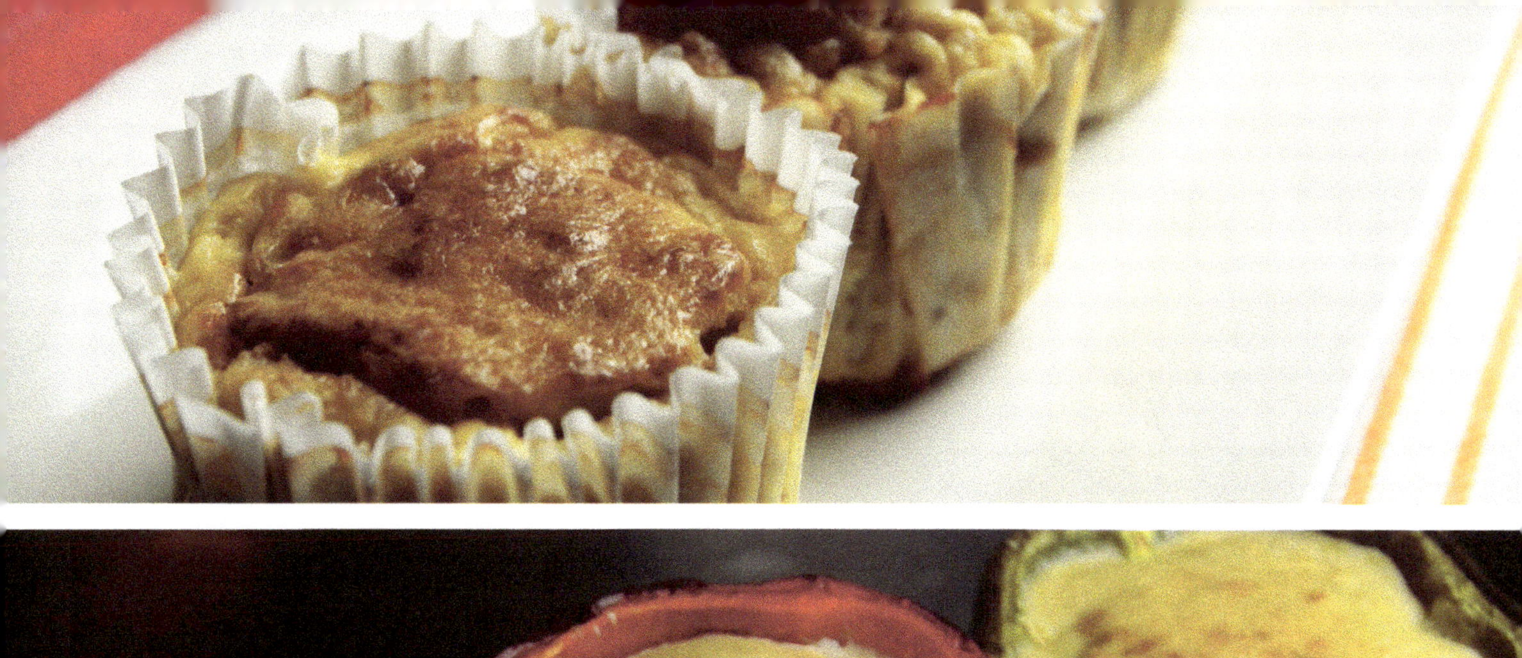

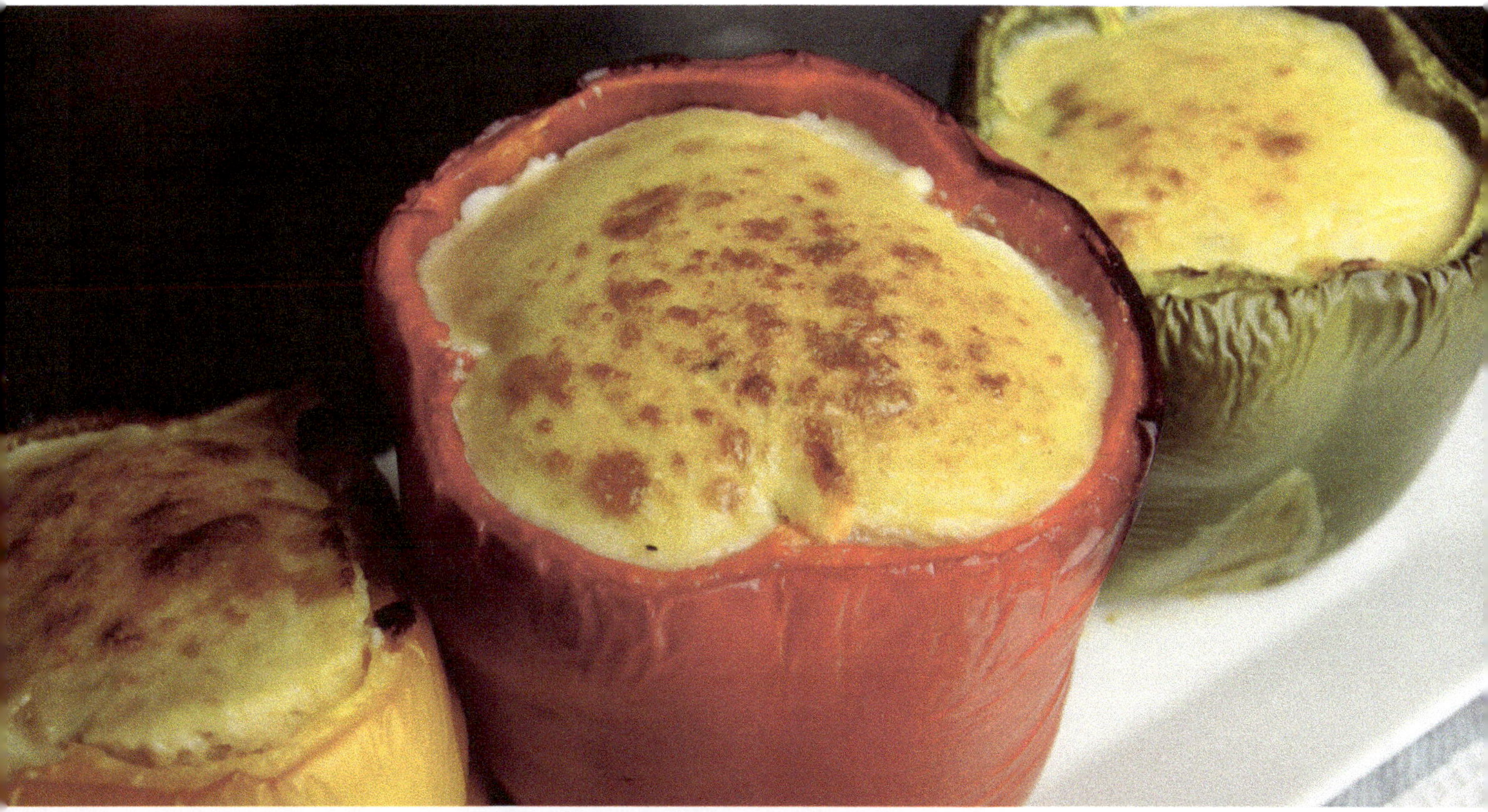

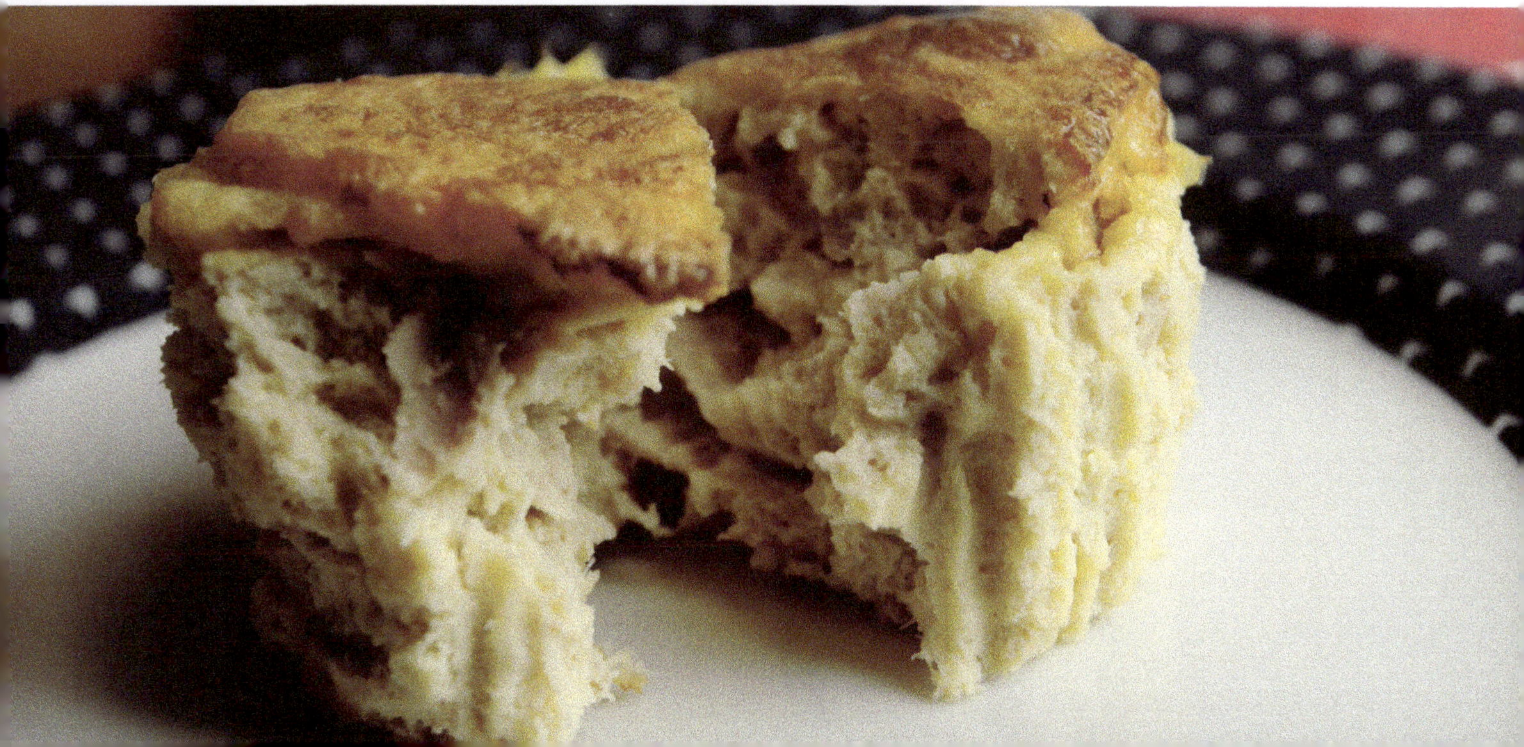

Almond Bread

Prep time: **15 min** - Cook time: **30 mins** - Servings: **5 to 6 (10 to 12 slices)**

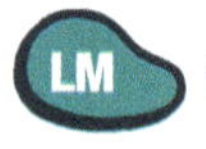

and

- 6 fresh eggs

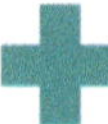

Ingredients:

- 2 ½ cups almond flour
- ¼ cup ground flaxseed
- 1 tablespoon extra-virgin olive oil
- 1 tablespoon vinegar
- 1 tablespoon fresh sage leaves, chopped
- 1 tablespoon fresh rosemary, chopped
- ½ teaspoon baking soda
- ½ teaspoon salt
- ***Optional:*** *1 large banana, mashed (200g)*

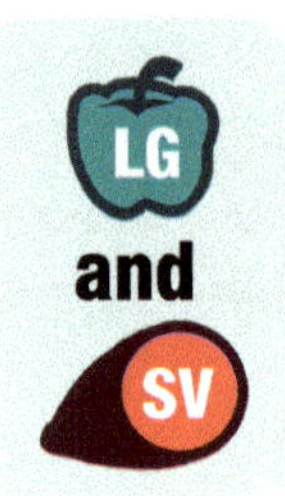

Method:

1. Preheat the oven to 180° / 360°F
2. Put the almond flour, flax seed, baking soda, salt and herbs in a bowl, and combine with an egg beater until mixed
3. Add the eggs, oil and vinegar. Mix again with an egg beater until well combined into a thick mixture. If you are also adding banana, add it here and mix in
4. Lightly brush the inside of a medium sized bread pan with olive oil. Dust the oil with a thin layer of almond flour. This will help the bread to not stick to the pan
5. Scoop the mixture into the pan and bake for 30 minutes, or until a toothpick comes out clean from the centre. Remove from oven, cover and let cool for 30 minutes

Recipe tips:

- *Cut into 10 to 12 slices so you have 2 slices per day*
- *This bread is very dense, so each slice is equivalent to around 2 normal bread slices. A favourite is to enjoy with butter, cheese and Vegemite or Marmite for a super simple and tasty breakfast. You can also toast it for extra flavour*
- *For a more hearty breakfast (and if you have the time), you can eat it topped with bacon and a fried egg*
- *Whatever your choice of topping, take care to avoid anything with sugar in it such as jam or Nutella, because the combination of sugar and fat will go straight to your hips!*

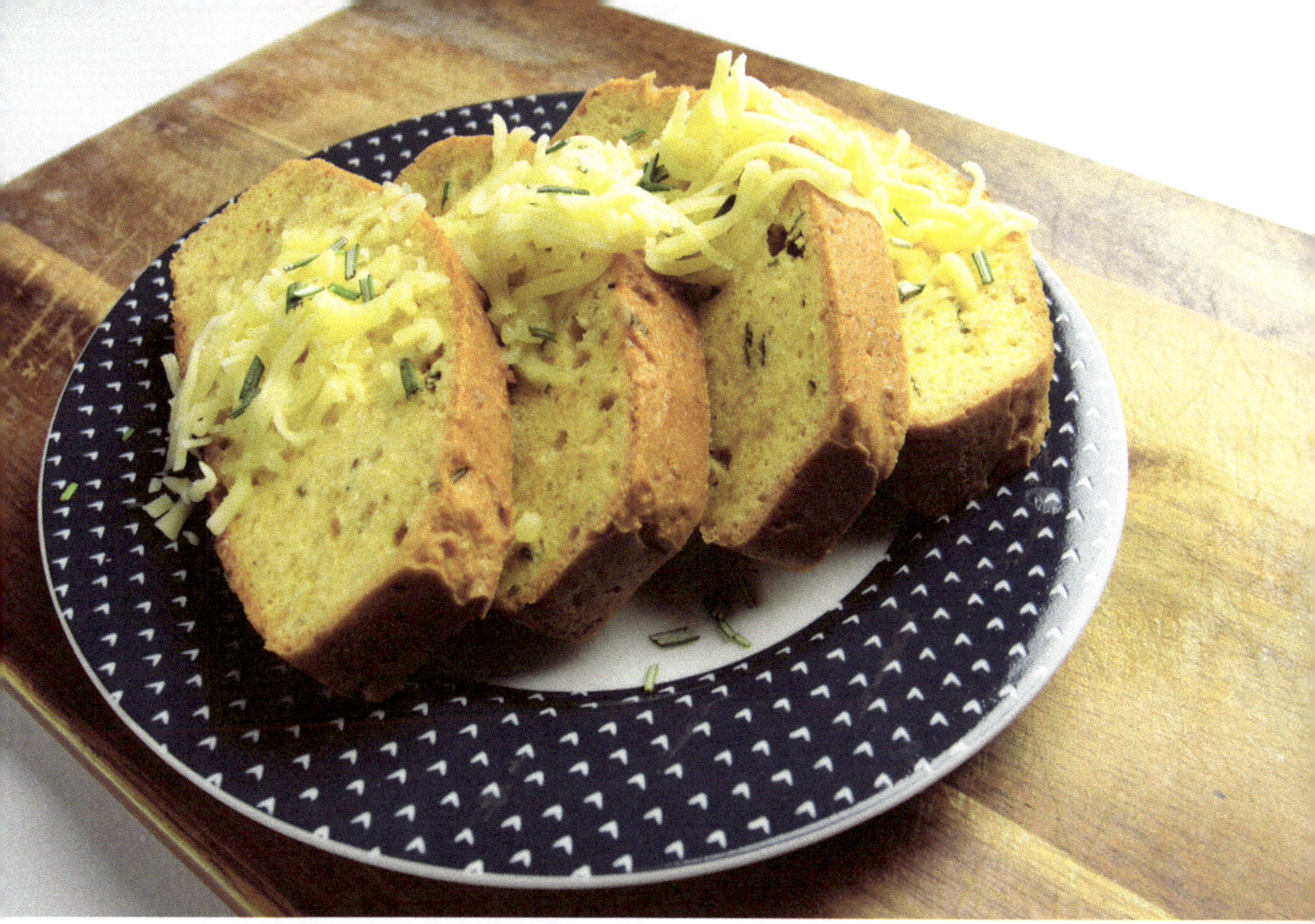

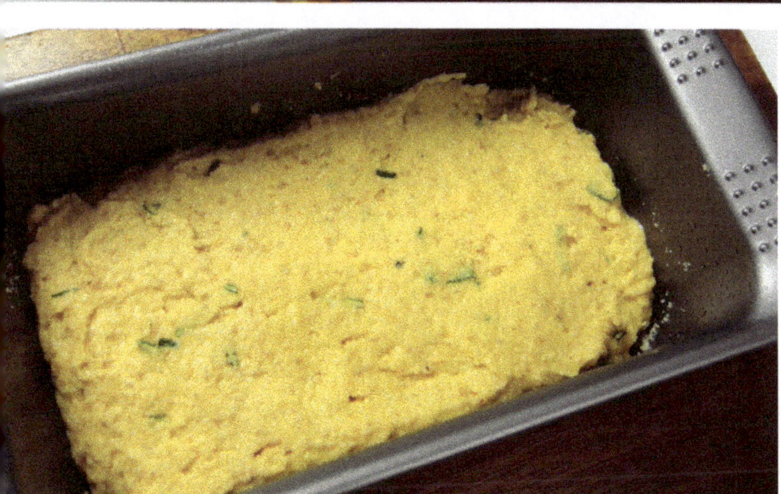
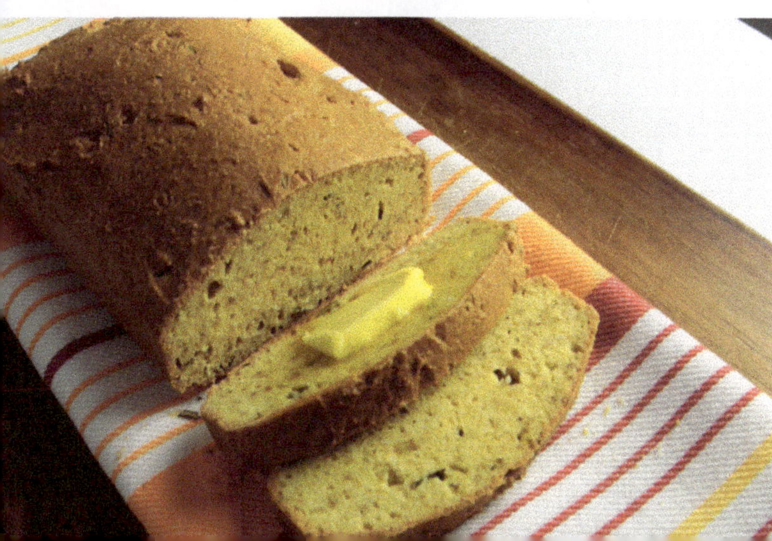
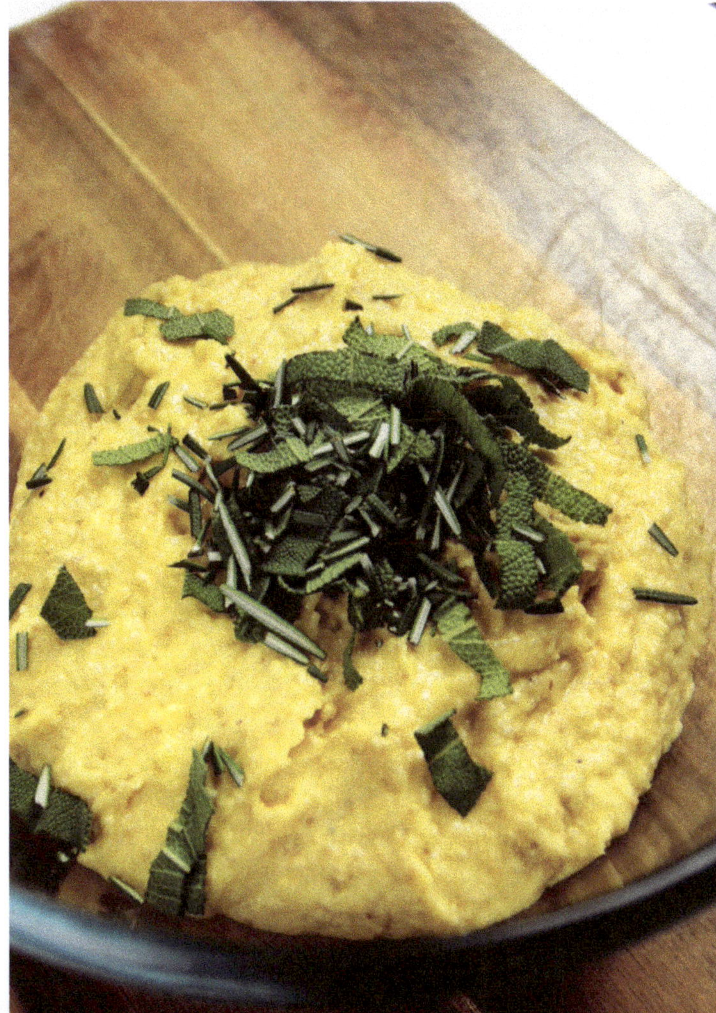

Chilli Con Sus

Prep time: ***25 mins*** *- Cook time:* ***1 to 1.5 hours*** *- Servings:* ***6 portions***

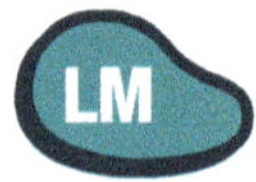

Lean meats

- 1.2 kg *low fat* beef, pork or chicken mince

OR

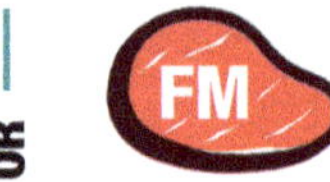

Fatty meats

- 1.2 kg beef or pork mince

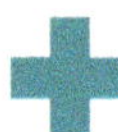

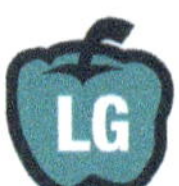

Low-GI veggies

- 4 carrots, diced
- 1 handful of spinach (per meal, to serve)
- 20g sour cream **OR** grated cheese (per meal, to serve)

OR

Starchy veggies

- 2 carrots, diced
- 100g mashed sweet potato **OR** pumpkin (per meal, to serve)
- 20g sour cream **OR** grated cheese (per meal, to serve)

OR

Whole grain

- 2 carrots, diced
- 1 cup of brown rice – instant rice is fine **OR** quinoa (per meal, to serve)

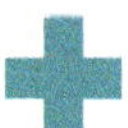

Other ingredients:

- 2 x 400g cans diced tomatoes
- 2 tablespoons of tomato paste
- 2 x 400g cans red kidney beans OR black beans OR chickpeas, drained and rinsed
- 4 sticks of celery, chopped
- 2 large onions, finely chopped
- 1 red capsicum, peeled and diced
- 3 chillies finely chopped (choose a variety with the right level of heat for you)
- 8 garlic cloves, crushed
- 1 tablespoon coconut oil
- 2 cups beef stock or water

Mexican chilli powder mix

- 2 teaspoons ground coriander
- 2 teaspoons ground cumin
- 2 teaspoons ground chilli powder
- 2 teaspoons sweet smoked paprika
- 2 teaspoons dried oregano
- 1 teaspoon dried onion
- 2 bay leaves
- pinch of salt and pepper (to taste)

Method:

1. Heat oil in a large saucepan over medium heat. Add onions and cook for 5 minutes until translucent. Add mince and fry, stirring with a spoon to break up mince until browned
2. Add Mexican Chilli Powder mix and cook, stirring, until fragrant and the mince is coated
3. Add in all vegetables - capsicum, garlic, celery, carrots and the chopped chilli. Cook for 5 to 10 minutes or until vegetables are just starting to soften
4. Pour in the tomatoes, tomato paste, bay leaves and beef stock or water (the liquid should just about cover the mince mixture). Bring to the boil then reduce heat. Partially cover the saucepan and simmer for 30-40 minutes
5. Now add in the kidney beans and cook for about 15 minutes to let the beans heat through and the liquid reduce. You may want to turn the heat up a little if the liquid isn't reducing
6. Season with salt and pepper to taste

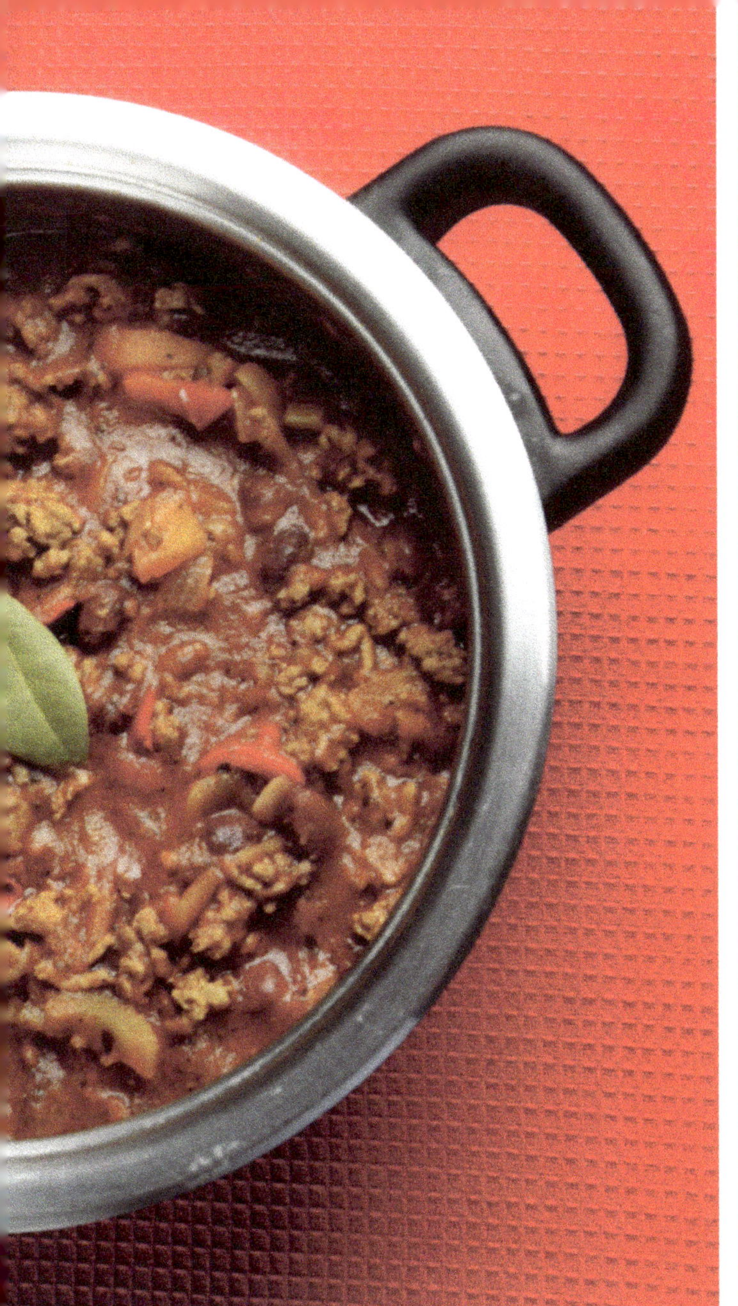

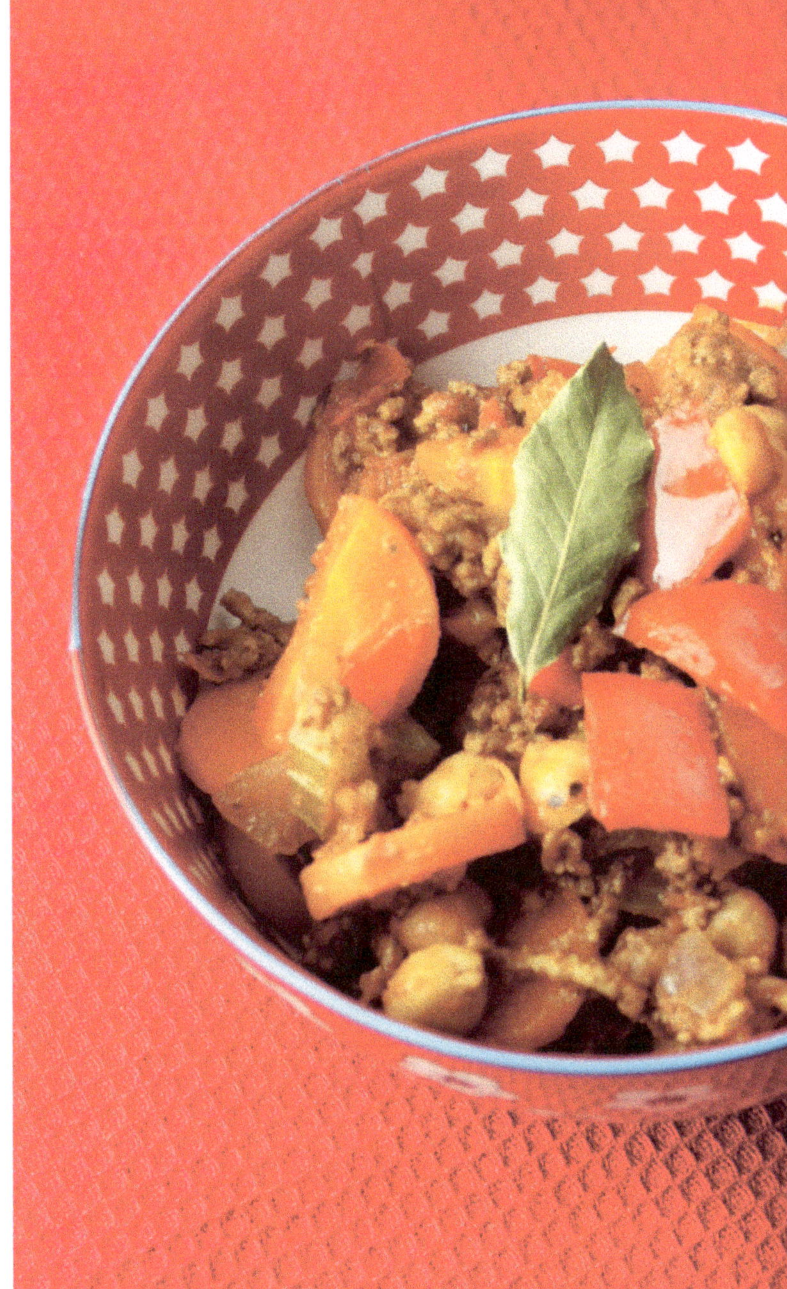

Recipe tips:

- *The vegetables and beans in this chilli means you can eat it as a complete meal, or you can serve over other foods as indicated by the meal plans (sweet potato, brown rice, and so on)*
- *You can vary the recipe by using different meats and different vegetables, and also by experimenting with various herb and spice mixtures*
- *One big saucepan will make the recipe easier to manage, though if you don't have a big enough pot, you can get two going at the same time*
- *Save time on chopping by using a food processor. It will save you heaps of time in the long run, so definitely worth the investment!*
- *Chilli Con Sus keeps well in an airtight container in the fridge for up to a week. Alternatively, try freezing flat in freezer bags. Freezing flat means you can stack the frozen bags easily in your freezer, the food will defrost quickly and you can snap off one portion without defrosting the rest*

Turkey Burgers

Prep time: **20 min** - Cook time: **10-15 mins** - Servings: **6 to 8**

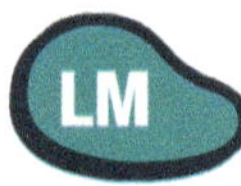

Lean meats

- 1kg lean chicken or beef mince
- 4 fresh eggs

OR

Fatty meats

- 1kg turkey mince
- 8 pieces of bacon
- 4 fresh eggs

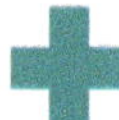

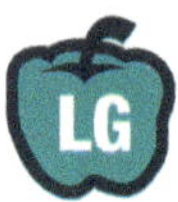

Low-GI veggies

- 1 head of iceberg lettuce – Cut off pieces to use in place of buns **OR** eat with 100g of frozen low-GI veggies

OR

Starchy veggies

- Cut 2 cm (1 inch) discs of a large sweet potato (100g per serving). Bake at 200° / 400°F for 10 mins, turn and another 10 mins

OR

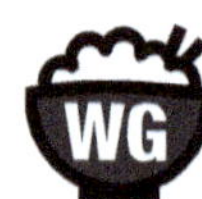

Whole grain

- Eat with a rye bread bun **OR** break up and eat with 1 cup of brown rice and Avo dressing

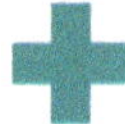

Ingredients:

- 2 carrots, grated (300g)
- 3 zucchinis, grated (500g)
- 4 eggs
- 3 cloves of garlic, finely chopped
- 2 tablespoons of virgin coconut oil
- 1 small brown onion, finely diced
- Salt and pepper to taste

Avo dressing

- 1 large ripe avocado
- 1 tablespoon dried dill
- 1 tablespoon Dijon mustard
- ½ cup skim milk
- Salt and pepper

Place all ingredients in a food processor and combine till a smooth dressing consistency is achieved. Add more spices and water until you reach the desired consistency.

Method:

1. Fry the onion (and bacon if included) in a frying pan on high heat with butter until it turns slightly brown
2. Mix all the ingredients together. Roll in tight balls, take care to press all ingredients firmly together to ensure meatballs don't fall apart during cooking. Flatten into patties
3. Cook on a barbeque over medium heat for about 5 minutes on each side, or until cooked through. Or cook in a pan over medium heat for the same amount of time

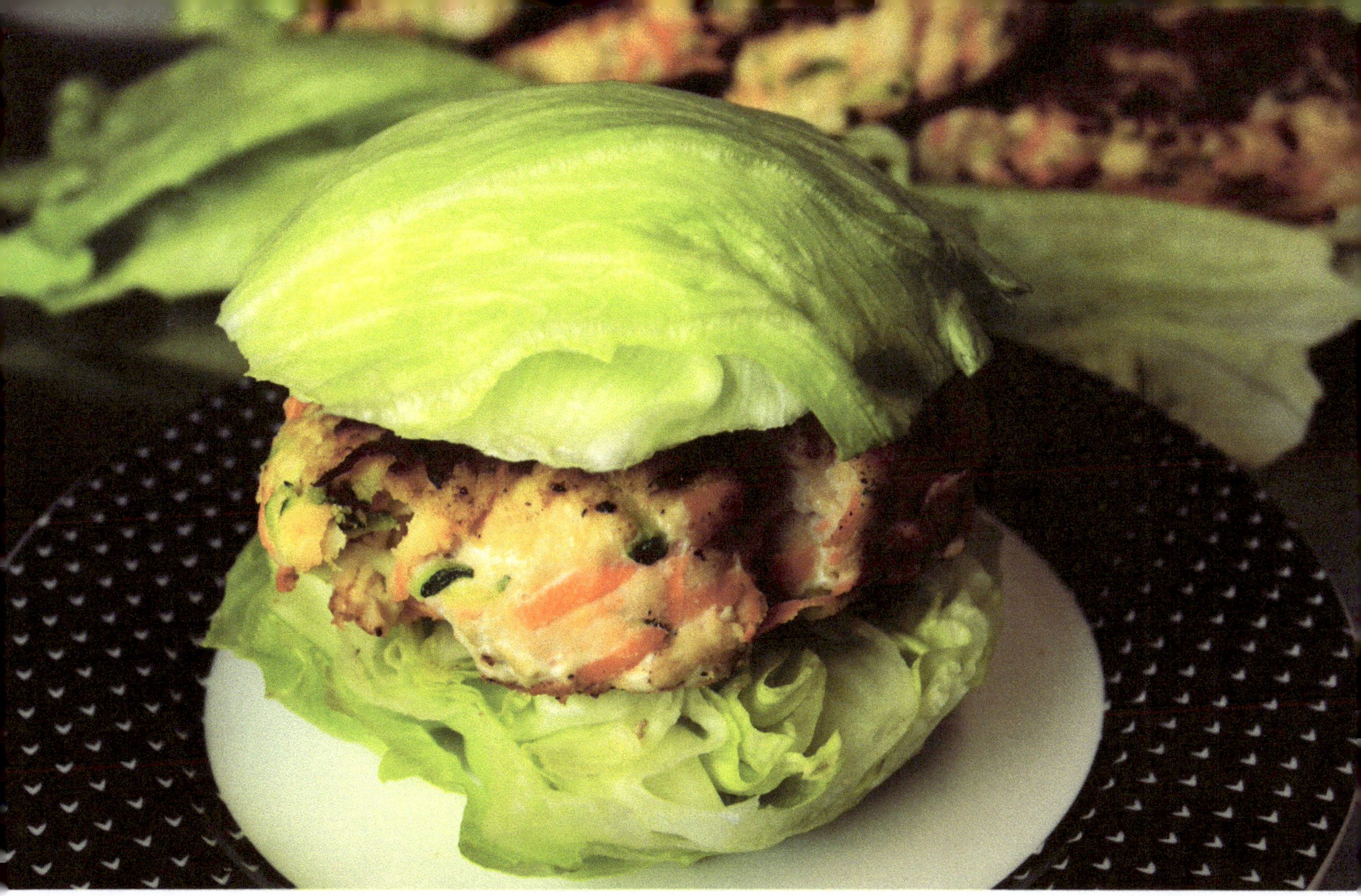

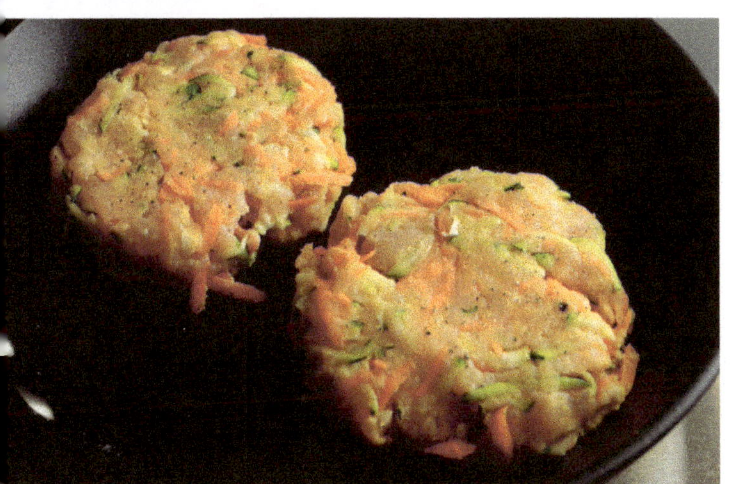

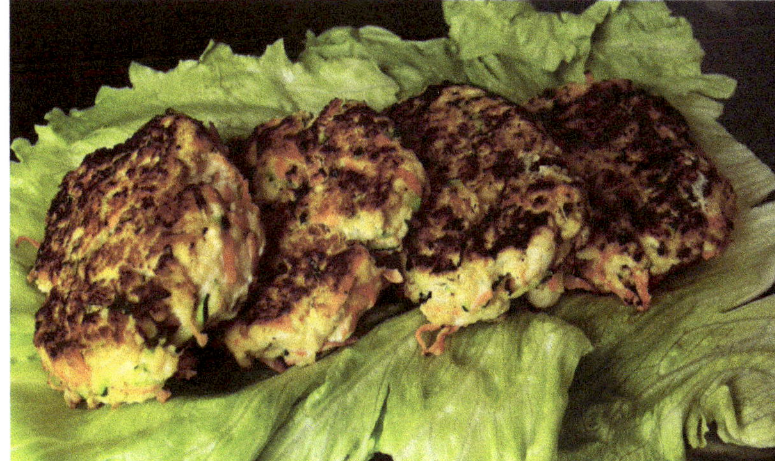

Recipe tips:

- *If cooking on a stove top, get two pans going so that you can cook them faster*
- *You can also bake them all at once in the oven – try 10 mins on 200° /* 400°F, and check when it is cooked through
- *These burgers are very versatile as you can eat them on their own, or make burgers out of them with various other foods (like lettuce, sweet potato, or buns). They're a great backup to have in the freezer when you need something easy and healthy.*
- *Save time on chopping by using a food processor. It will save you heaps of time in the long run, so definitely worth the investment!*

Fast Chicken Bake

Prep time: **10 mins** - Cook time: **35 mins** - Servings: **6 to 7**

Lean meats

- 1.5kg chicken breast, butterflied

OR

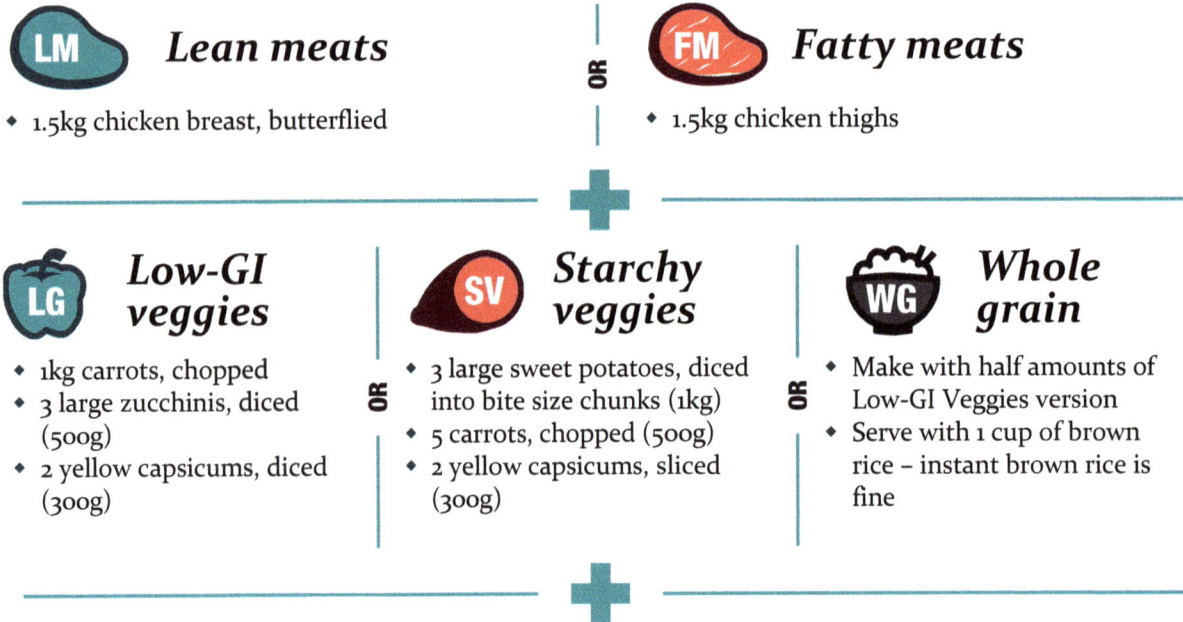

Fatty meats

- 1.5kg chicken thighs

Low-GI veggies

- 1kg carrots, chopped
- 3 large zucchinis, diced (500g)
- 2 yellow capsicums, diced (300g)

OR

Starchy veggies

- 3 large sweet potatoes, diced into bite size chunks (1kg)
- 5 carrots, chopped (500g)
- 2 yellow capsicums, sliced (300g)

OR

Whole grain

- Make with half amounts of Low-GI Veggies version
- Serve with 1 cup of brown rice – instant brown rice is fine

Spice options:

Pick one of these spice options to mix up the bake.

Spices for the vegetables

- 1 teaspoon oregano
- ½ teaspoon parsley
- ½ teaspoon dried mint leaves

Spices for the chicken

- ½ teaspoon paprika
- ¼ teaspoon thyme
- Salt and pepper to taste

Chimichurri marinade

- 1 bunch flat leaf parsley
- 2 shallots, diced
- 2 garlic cloves, crushed
- 2 chillies, diced (seeds removed)
- juice of one lemon
- zest of half lemon
- 2 tablespoons red wine vinegar
- 1 tablespoon extra-virgin olive oil
- Salt and pepper

Place all ingredients into a blender and process until blended. Coat chicken with marinade before placing on vegetables

Oriental Marinade

- 2 shallots, diced
- 2 garlic cloves, crushed
- 2 chillies, diced (seeds removed)
- 1 tablespoon fresh ginger, chopped
- 1 bunch coriander
- 1 bunch mint leaves
- 1 tablespoon extra-virgin olive oil
- 2 tablespoons rice wine vinegar
- Juice of half a lime
- 1 tablespoon fish sauce
- 1 teaspoon soy sauce

Place all ingredients into a blender and process until blended. Coat chicken with marinade before placing on vegetables

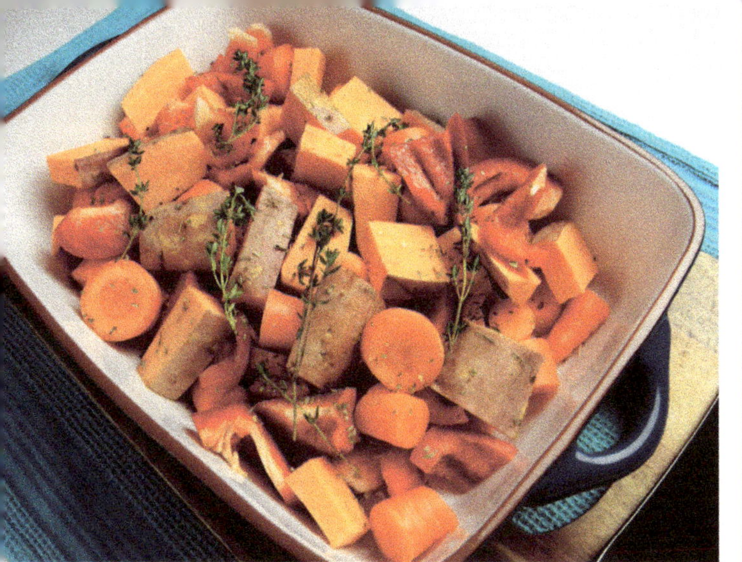

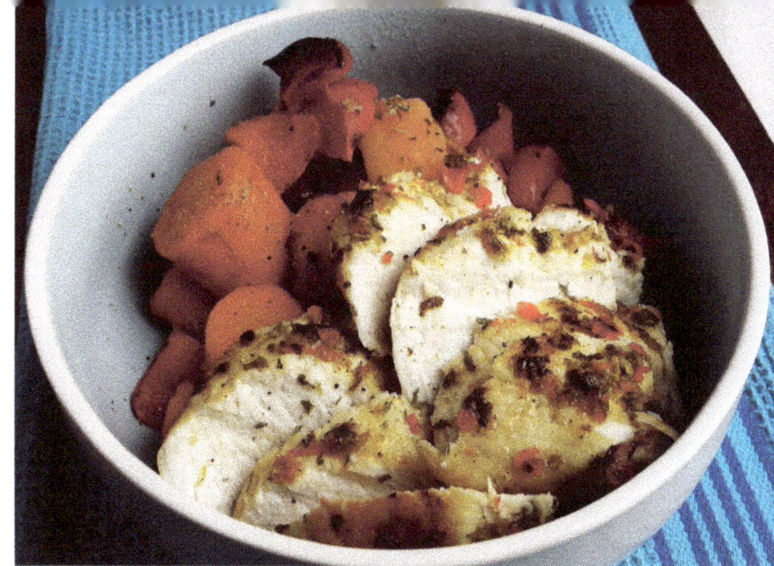

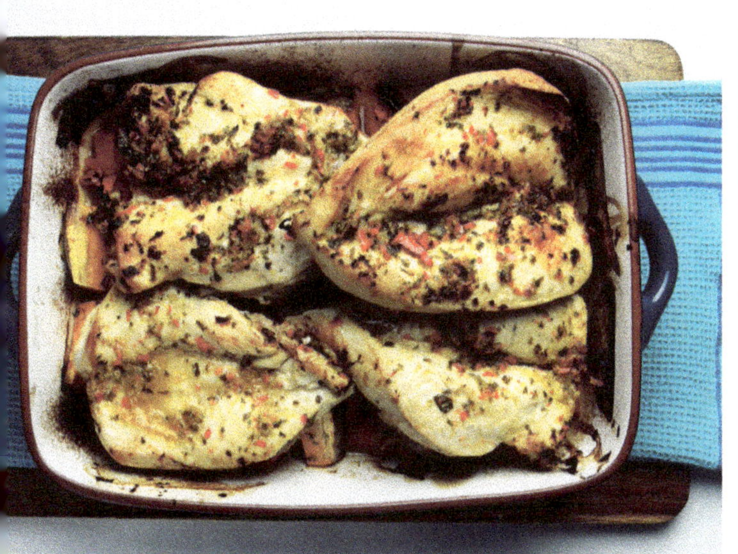

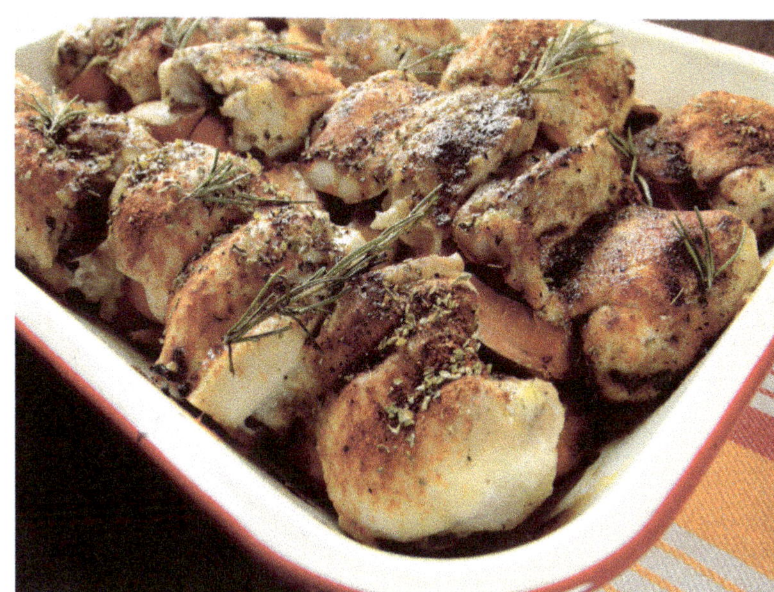

Method:

1. Preheat the oven to 180° / 360°F
2. Line a large baking tray with foil, or coat inside lightly with extra virgin olive oil
3. Spread the vegetables evenly on the foil and top with oregano, parsley and mint. If adding broccoli, place it at the bottom to protect from direct heat
4. Place in oven for 20 minutes
5. Lay chicken on top of the hot vegetables. Coat with paprika and thyme if not using a marinade
6. Cook for another 30 mins or until the chicken is cooked through
7. Remove and drain liquid from the tray. Divide into meals for the week and store in freezer bags

Recipe notes:

- *You can skip baking vegetables altogether and just bake the chicken on its own. That way you can combine with different frozen vegetables each day for more variety and you'll be saving even more time*
- *You can easily make the recipe with up to 1.5kg chicken at once. My small oven handles it well and provides additional meals for the week. Just add more vegetables alongside and make sure you have a big enough pan*
- *If eating with rice, save some of the cooking juices as gravy to spice up the rice*

Beef Stew

Prep time: **20 mins** - Cook time: **4 hours** - Servings: 6 - 7

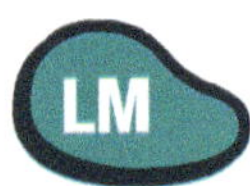

Lean meats

- 1.5kg lean beef cuts, diced

OR

Fatty meats

- 1.5kg lamb, pork or other beef cuts, diced

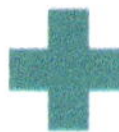

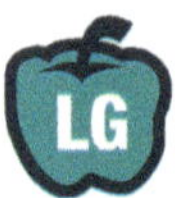

Low-GI veggies

- 500g squash, sliced
- 500g mushrooms, chopped
- 3 carrots, sliced (300g)
- 1 brown onion, chopped

OR

Starchy veggies

- 1kg sweet potato, chopped into chunks
- 3 carrots, sliced (300g)
- 1 brown onion, chopped

OR

Whole grain

- Make with half amounts of Low-GI Veggies version
- Serve with 1 cup of brown rice – instant brown rice is fine **OR** serve with rye bread

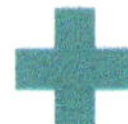

Spice options:

Pick one of these spice options to mix up the bake.

Traditional stew

- 1 cup parsley, chopped
- 2 tablespoons dried mint
- ½ cup coconut flour
- 3 cups boiling water
- 3 beef stock cubes
- 2 tablespoons tomato paste
- Salt and pepper to taste

Spanish Stew

- 2 tablespoons sweet paprika
- 1 tablespoon cumin
- 1 teaspoon dried chilli
- ½ cup coconut flour
- 3 cups boiling water
- 3 beef stock cubes
- 2 tablespoons tomato paste
- Salt and pepper to taste

Fresh herb mix

- 4 sprigs fresh rosemary
- 2 sprigs fresh thyme
- ½ cup fresh mint
- 2 sprigs fresh oregano
- ½ cup coconut flour
- 3 cups boiling water
- 3 beef stock cubes
- 2 tablespoons tomato paste
- Salt and pepper to taste

Chop fresh herbs and cover meat before adding to the stew

Method:

1. Preheat the oven to 130° / 270°F
2. Coat diced meat with flour and set aside. Save the remaining flour
3. In a large baking pan, place half the vegetables in a layer, topped with half of the meat, and repeat layers with remaining vegetables and meat
4. Mix the boiling water with remaining flour, tomato paste and spices. If there is no flour left after coating the meat, add a tablespoon of coconut flour
5. Pour into the baking pan, stopping when the mixture just covers the ingredients. Add more boiling water if needed. Cover and cook for 4 hours, or until the sauce has thickened
6. Divide into meals and freeze

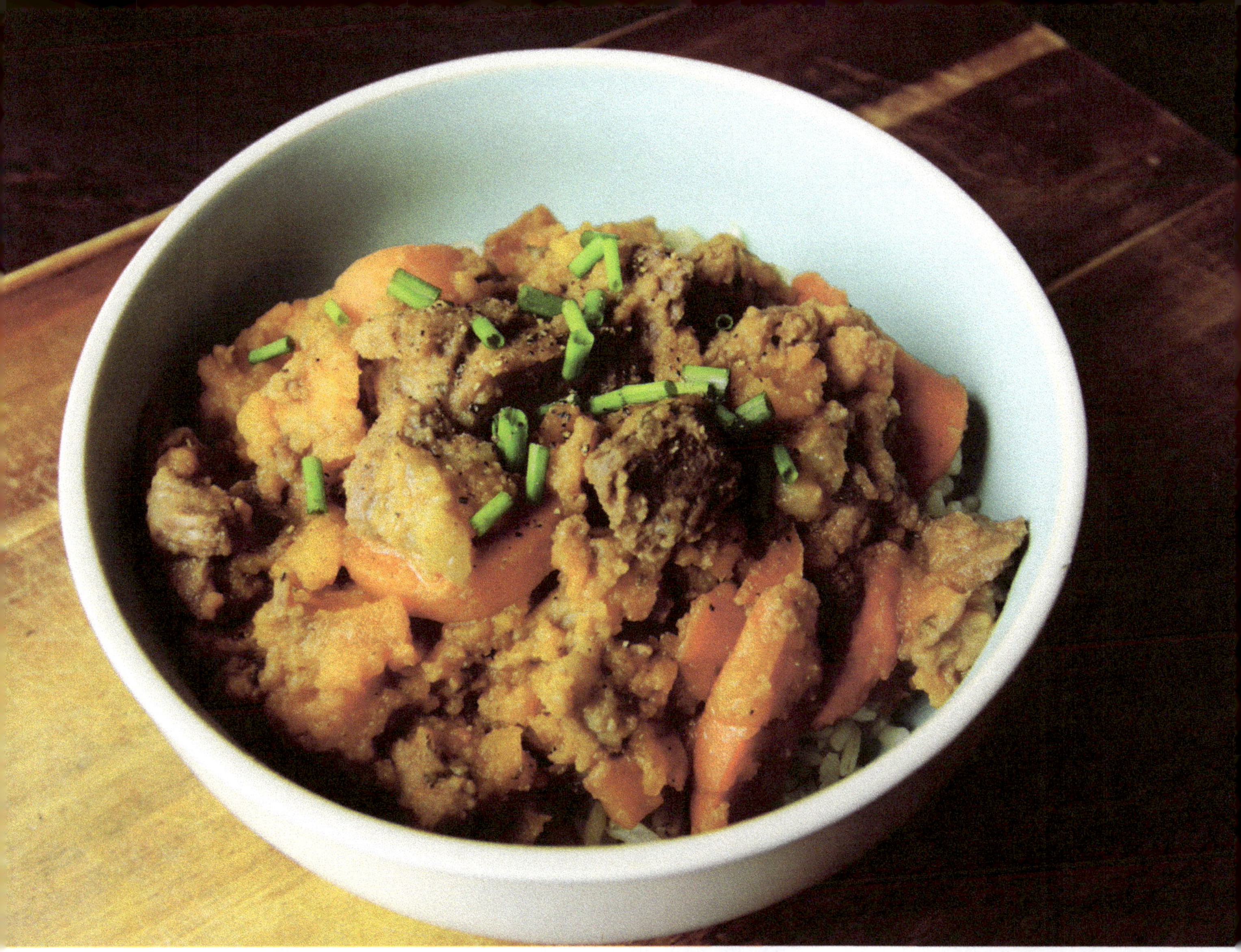

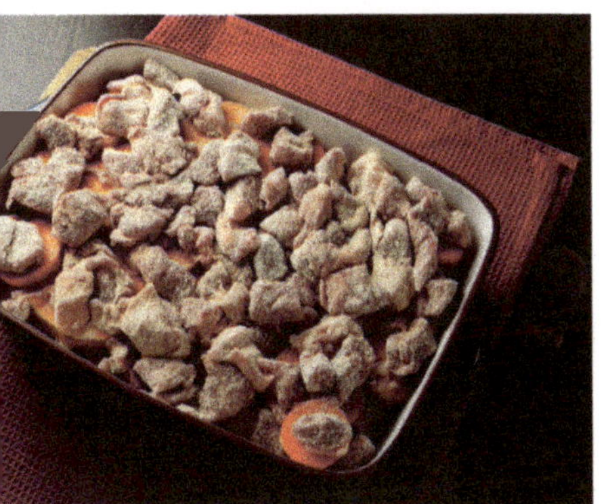

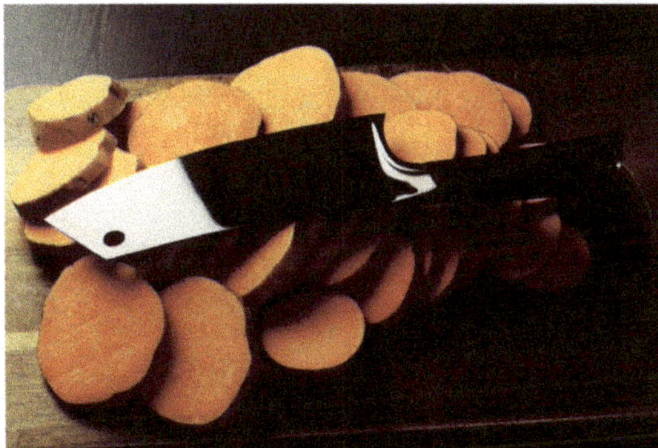

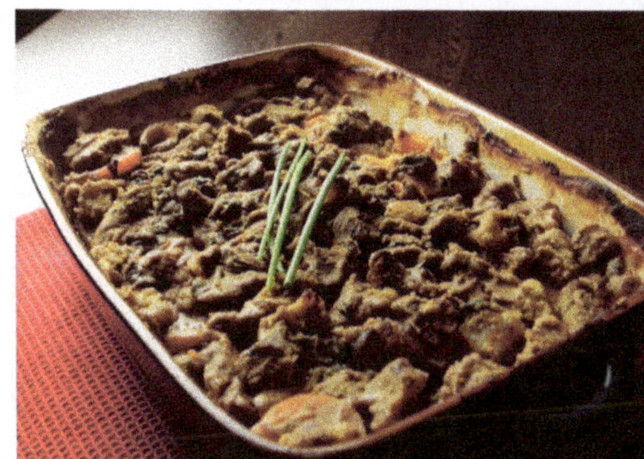

Recipe notes:

- *This is a very scalable dish, so you can easily make a larger version for more meals or to feed more people. Just check at the end of cooking that the meat is tender and sauce is thick*
- *When including grains, simply add a cup of brown rice or quinoa. You can also eat with a whole wheat pasta, though brown rice is a healthier choice*
- *You can also try with lamb, pork or chicken. Mix it up to keep it interesting!*

Lamb Roast

Prep time: **10 mins** - Cook time: **35 mins** - Servings: **6 to 7**

Lean meats

- 1.5kg lamb **OR** beef shoulder, fat removed and butterflied

OR

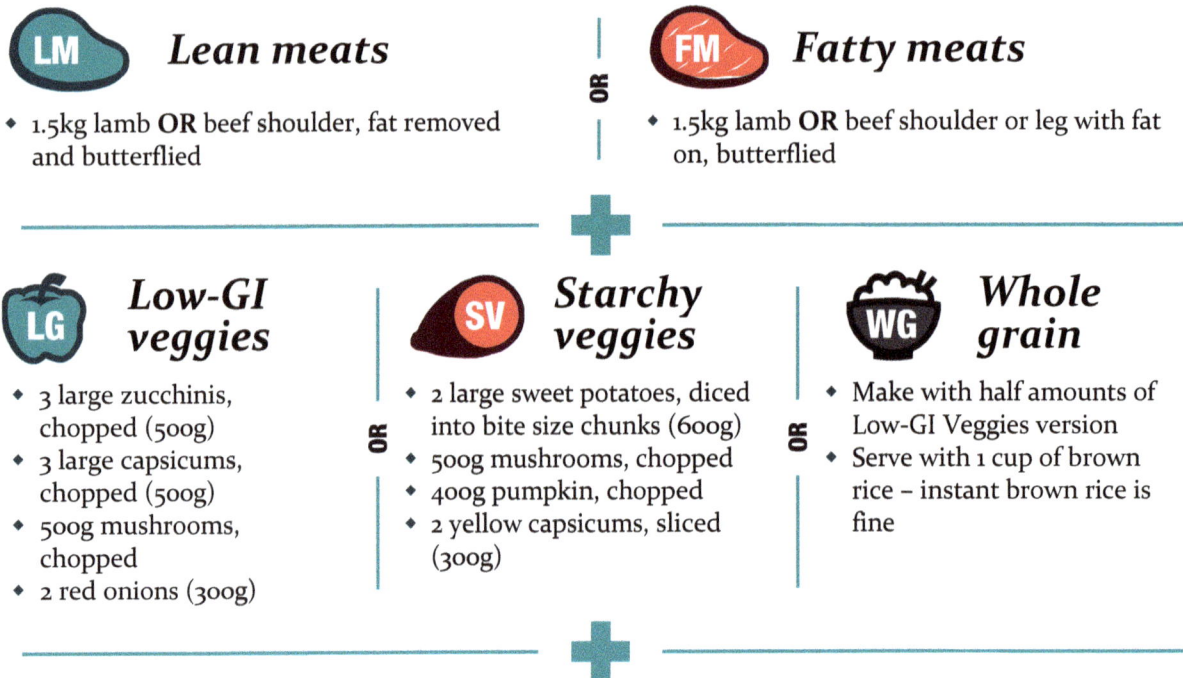

Fatty meats

- 1.5kg lamb **OR** beef shoulder or leg with fat on, butterflied

Low-GI veggies

- 3 large zucchinis, chopped (500g)
- 3 large capsicums, chopped (500g)
- 500g mushrooms, chopped
- 2 red onions (300g)

OR

Starchy veggies

- 2 large sweet potatoes, diced into bite size chunks (600g)
- 500g mushrooms, chopped
- 400g pumpkin, chopped
- 2 yellow capsicums, sliced (300g)

OR

Whole grain

- Make with half amounts of Low-GI Veggies version
- Serve with 1 cup of brown rice – instant brown rice is fine

Pick your flavour:

Spices for the vegetables

- 1 teaspoon oregano
- ½ teaspoon parsley
- ½ teaspoon dried mint leaves

Spices for a sweet potato mix

- 1 teaspoon sweet paprika
- ½ teaspoon cumin
- ¼ teaspoon salt

Rosemary Mint Marinade

- 5 whole sprigs fresh rosemary
- 40g dried rosemary
- 10 leaves fresh mint
- ¼ teaspoon dried onion
- ¼ teaspoon garlic
- 1 tablespoon extra-virgin olive oil
- ¼ teaspoon salt

Place all ingredients except the whole rosemary sprigs into a blender and process until blended. Coat roast with blend. Make five cuts along the roast and place fresh sprigs inside (as shown)

Mustard Marinade

- 2 tablespoons rosemary
- 2 tablespoons dijon mustard
- 2 tablespoons extra virgin olive oil
- 1 tablespoon balsamic vinegar
- 1 tablespoon lemon juice
- 1 teaspoon black pepper
- 3 cloves garlic, minced
- 1 teaspoon salt

Mix all ingredients together, cover roast and marinade in fridge overnight

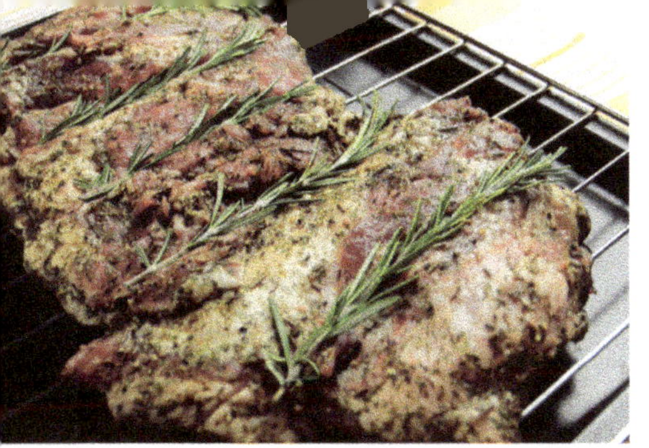

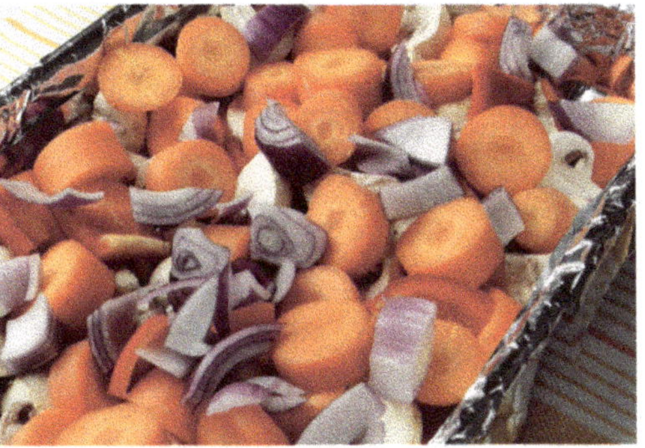

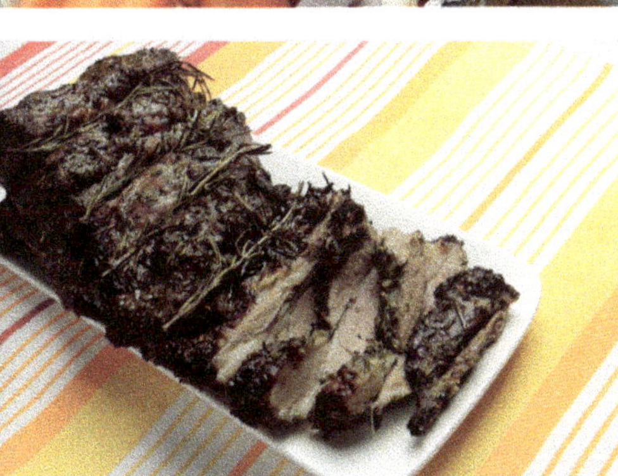

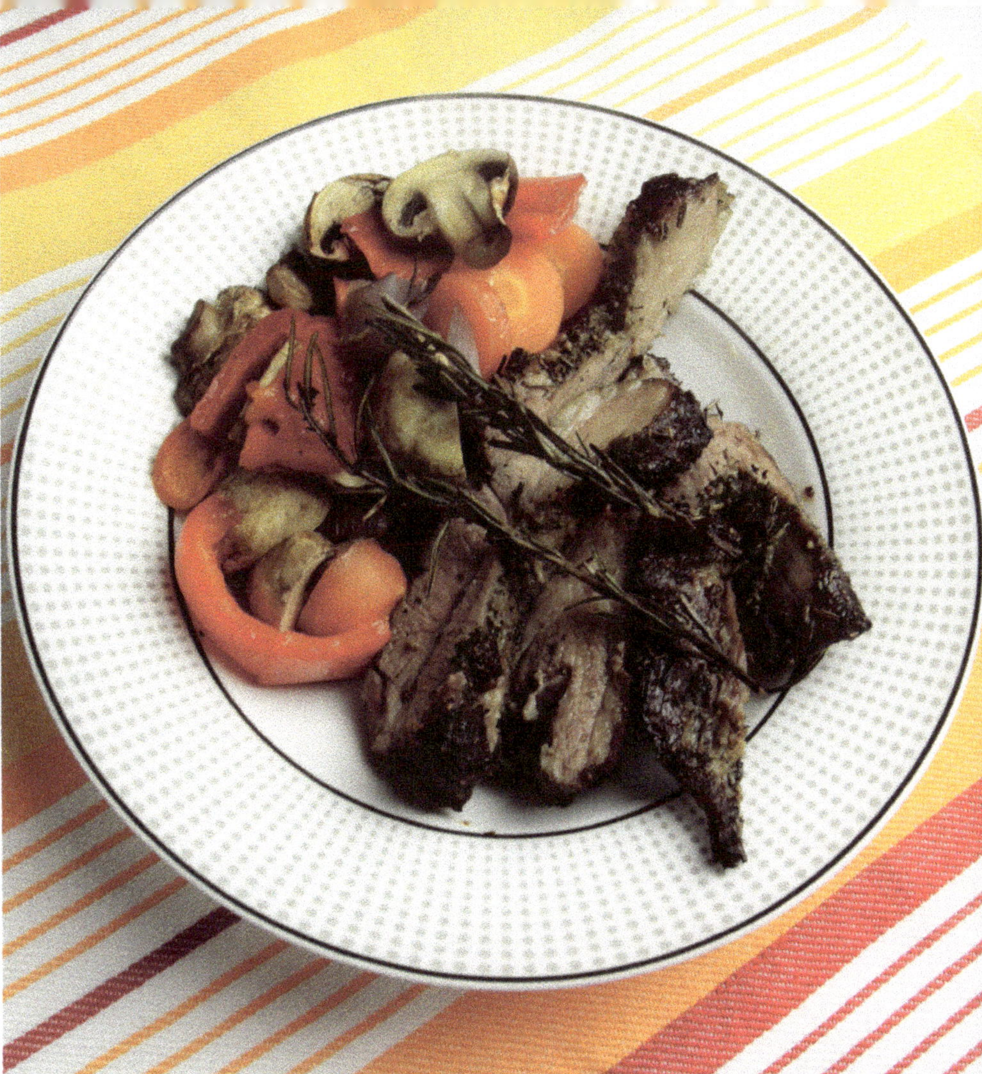

Method:

1. Preheat the oven to 180° / 360°F
2. Line a large baking tray with foil, or coat inside with extra virgin olive oil
3. Spread the vegetables evenly on the foil and top with your choice of herbs and spices. Place in the bottom of the oven
4. Place the roast on a grill tray above the vegetables in the oven so that the juices will drip down onto the vegetables
5. Cook for 30 to 35 mins or until the roast is cooked as desired
6. Remove the roast, cover with foil and let sit for 10 mins
7. Bake vegetables for another 10 minutes or until soft
8. Remove and drain liquid from the tray. Divide into meals for the week and store in freezer bags

Recipe notes:

- *Similar to the chicken bake, you can skip baking vegetables altogether and just bake the roast on its own. That way you can combine with different frozen vegetables each day for more variety and you'll be saving even more time*
- *If eating with rice, save some of the cooking juices as gravy to spice up the rice*

Anytime Meatballs

Prep time: **10 min** - Cook time: **15 mins** - Servings: **6**

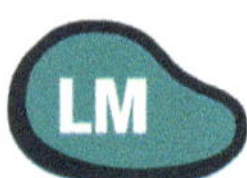

Lean meats

- 1.2kg lean beef **OR** chicken mince

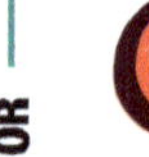

Fatty meats

- 1.2kg lamb **OR** beef **OR** pork mince

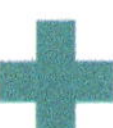

Meatballs

Ingredients:

- 2 tablespoons coconut oil
- 2 cloves garlic, crushed and chopped
- ½ red onion, chopped
- 2 egg yolks
- 1 teaspoon salt

Method:

1. Preheat the oven to 175° / 350°F
2. Mix all the ingredients together with the mince
3. With the palms of your hands, separate and roll into about 15 balls
4. Place in an oven-proof container and bake for 10 minutes or until cooked through
5. Turn over meatballs, add Fast Tomato Sauce to container and bake with lid on for another 5 minutes

Fast Tomato Sauce

This sauce is quick to make, but you can also substitute with store-bought, low-sugar or sugar-free pasta sauce.

Ingredients:

- 3 x 400g canned peeled tomatoes
- 1 tablespoon dried onion flakes (or fry diced onion)
- ½ teaspoon dried garlic (or fry 1 chopped garlic clove)
- 1 teaspoon oregano
- 1 teaspoon salt
- ½ teaspoon pepper

Method:

1. While the meatballs bake, combine all ingredients in a saucepan on medium heat for about 7 minutes or until it becomes a thick sauce

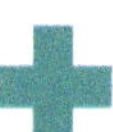

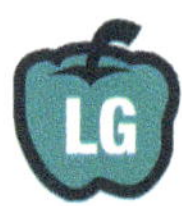

Low-GI veggies

- Your choice of steamed vegetable or salad mix
- Aim to get around 200g+ vegetables or salad in for each serve
- Peas, squash, asparagus, cauliflower, broccoli, onion, mushrooms

OR

Starchy veggies

- 3 large sweet potatoes, whole (1kg)

Line a baking tray with foil and place the sweet potatoes on top. Place on bottom tray so the meatballs can cook above. Bake potatoes for 45 minutes, remove from oven and remove peels. Mash and serve with meatballs

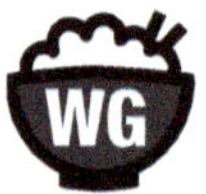

Whole grain

- Serve with 1 cup of brown rice – instant brown rice is fine **OR** 1 cup of cooked quinoa

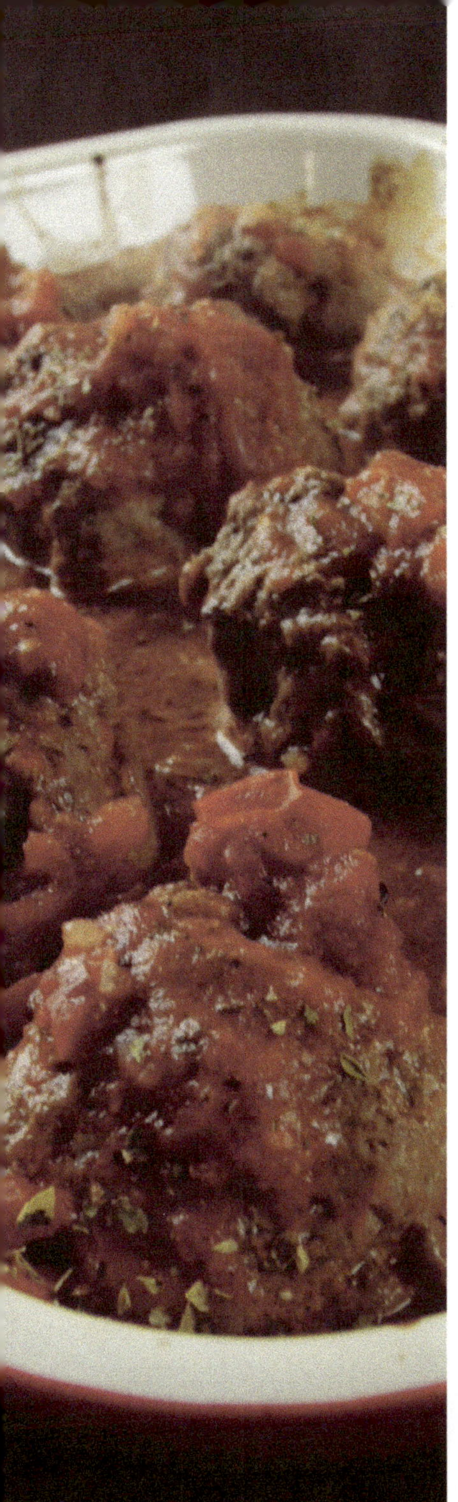
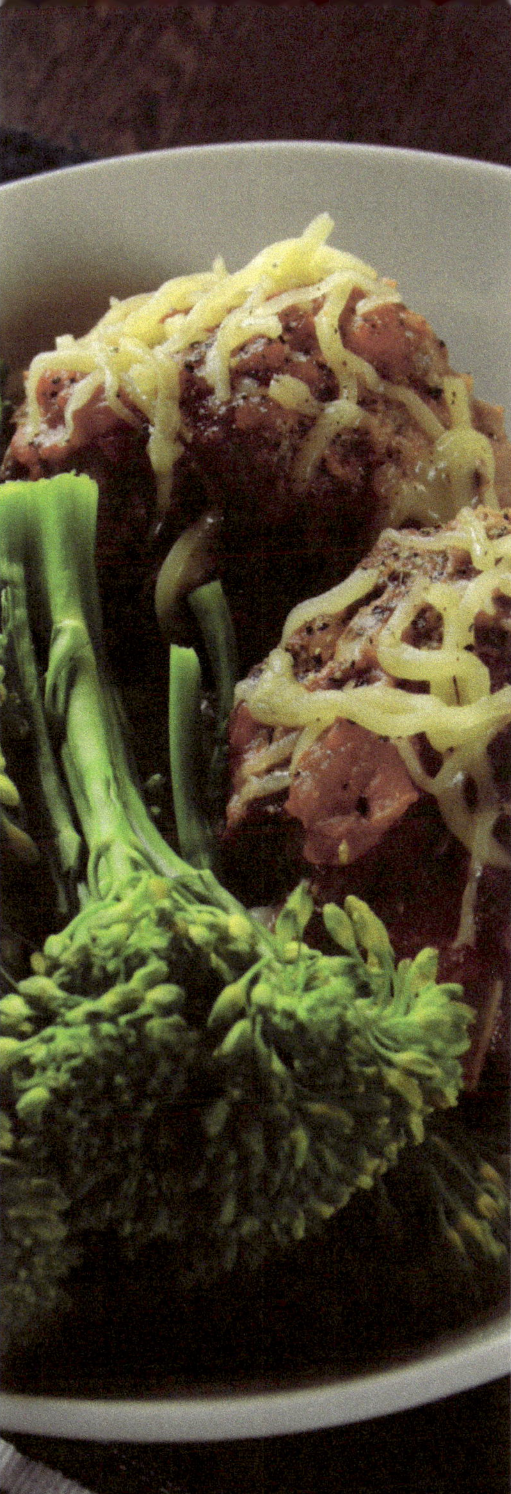
 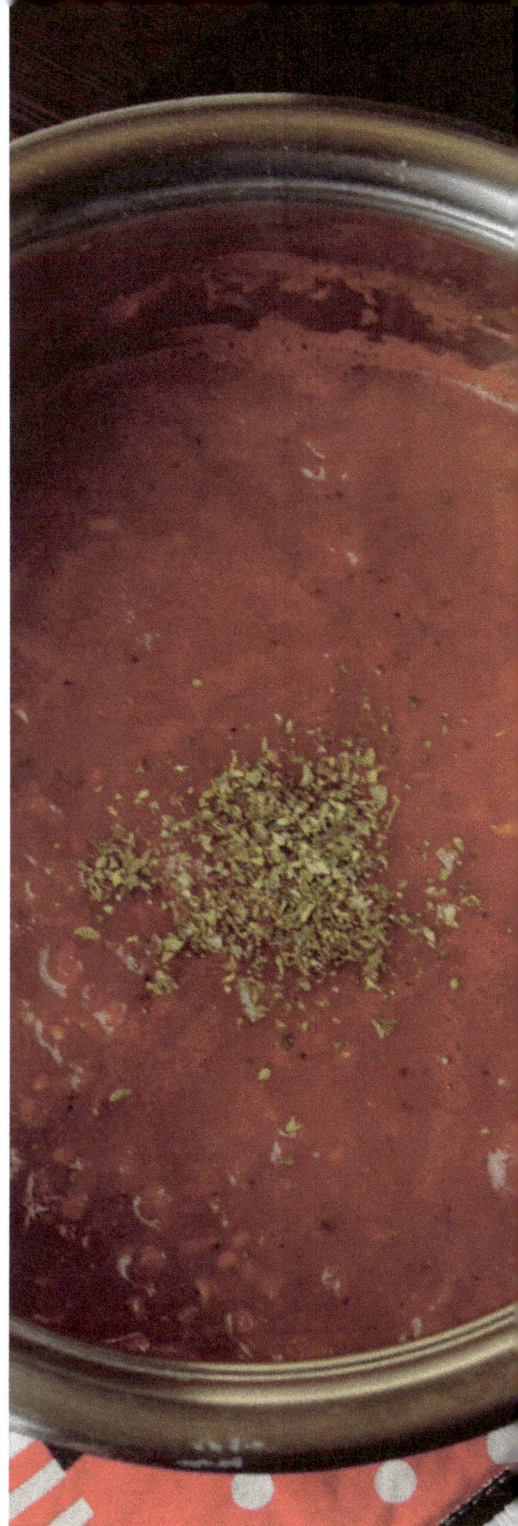

Recipe notes:

1. *Try using different meats such as lamb or pork to mix things up. Using lean beef can result in it drying out more quickly, so be careful not to overcook*
2. *Once you've divided these into containers, an easy option for low-GI vegetables is to add different kinds of frozen vegetables into the containers. Mixed steam bags can work really well, and allows you to mix it up between meals without any effort*
3. *For more zing in the meatballs, try adding a chilli to the sauce with a bit of cayenne pepper*
4. *Turn this into a bolognaise by putting all the ingredients into a saucepan and cook for 15 minutes*

Other bulk meal ideas

Each of the recipes above provide multiple options for variations. Beyond that you can turn almost any recipe into a bulk recipe by multiplying the ingredients. Here are a few other ideas you can try and adapt. Experiment and find what works for you!

Egg Salad

Prep time: **10 min** - Cook time: **15 to 40 mins** - Servings: **6**

Another easy breakfast-on-the-go is a simple hard-boiled egg salad. Easy to make and you can eat it anywhere!

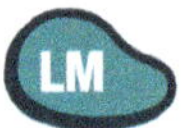

and

- 18 eggs (cook whole for 10 minutes in boiling water). Cool in cold water, peel and dice

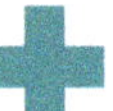

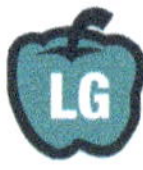

and

- 400g sweet tolanato **OR** cherry tomatoes, halved
- 400g English cucumbers, diced
- 150g sharp cheddar cheese, diced
- 1 head of lettuce, chopped

Method:

- Combine all ingredients as a salad. Serve with salsa or another sugar-free sauce if desired

Poached Chicken Salad

Prep time: **10 min** - Cook time: **1 to 1.5 hours** - Servings: **6**

Shredded chicken is super versatile and you can use it for a breakfast salad, a main meal or as a snack through the day. Poaching chicken is easy, or buying a roasted chicken is even easier!

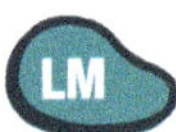

- Poach 1.5kg chicken breast (1.5 hours in boiling water with chicken stock)

- Poach 1.5kg chicken thigh (1 hour in boiling water with chicken stock)

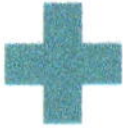

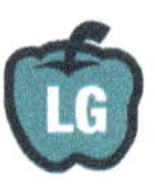

- Add 200g of a frozen low-GI vegetable mix with every portion

- Cook 1.5kg sweet potato to make mash

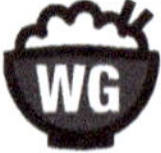

- Serve with a cup of brown rice **OR** 1 cup whole wheat pasta

Method:

- You can also buy a roasted chicken and shred the meat to save more time, but generally it's better to cook yourself
- If you'd like to add a sauce, use a sugar-free sauce like salsa for a salad or the Fast Tomato Sauce from the **Anytime Meatballs** recipe on **page 54** to eat with rice or sweet potato mash

Fish Galore

Prep time: **10 min** - Cook time: **15 to 40 mins** - Servings: **6**

Eating fish on a regular basis is a great boost to health because it's full of omega-3. Try this simple approach!

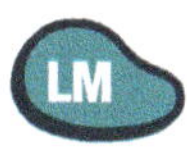 and 

- 1.5kg salmon with skin on (or your favourite fish, like cod or barramundi)

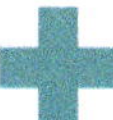

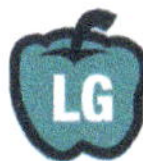

- 2kg mix of zucchini, broccolini and red capsicum

- 2kg mix of sweet potato, pumpkin and squash

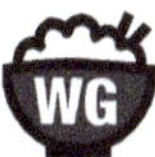

- 500g mushrooms
- 2 brown onion, diced
- Serve with a cup of brown rice

Method:

- Place the fish on a baking tray lined with foil and lightly grease with butter or olive oil
- Season with salt, pepper, rosemary, dill and lemon juice. Place a slice of lemon on each piece of fish
- Bake at 230° / 450°F for 12 to 15 minutes until fish is cooked but still juicy
- Below the fish you can place a baking pan with around 2kg vegetables. For softer vegetables like broccoli and zucchini, bake for 25 minutes. For hardy vegetables like carrots and sweet potato, bake for 40 minutes in total, or until soft

Bulk Bolognese

Prep time: **10 min** - Cook time: **25 mins** - Servings: **6**

Skip all the fuss and just make a simple Bolognese with off the shelf products.

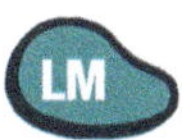

- 1.5kg low fat beef **OR** chicken mince

- 1.5kg beef **OR** lamb **OR** pork mince

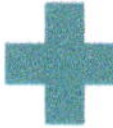

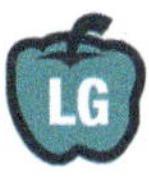

- Add 200g of a frozen low-GI vegetable mix with every portion

- Cook 1.5kg sweet potato to make mash

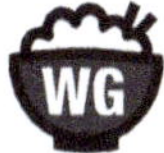

- Serve with a cup of brown rice **OR** 1 cup whole wheat pasta

Method:

- Cook 1.5kg mince in a large wok until brown
- Add 1 litre of no-sugar or low-sugar Bolognese sauce in and simmer for 10 minutes
- Divide and freeze portions. Serve with grated parmesan or mozzarella cheese

Get Fit To Get Lean

4 Workouts

Nutrition controls your weight, while the type and amount of exercise you do controls body composition. When we talk about body composition, we mean the ratio and amount of muscle mass to body fat. Knowing your target body type means you have a general idea of the kind of body composition that you want and the kind of exercise you should do to attain it. To help you get there, this book will give you fast and efficient workouts so you can fit exercise into your busy lifestyle.

We will cover four workout routines. Each of the routines are between 15 to 25 minutes, and are designed so that you can do them at home. These factors drastically reduce the amount of time you need to invest into workouts each week since you don't have to prepare and drive to a gym, and rather than spend an hour each time, you can easily do a quick 20 minutes in the morning before going to work or when you get home. This is also a great way to save money as you don't need a gym membership and need very little equipment to get started.

Now you can really see the beauty of these workouts – you save time and money, while still getting the great lean and healthy body you want! We're not cutting corners, but instead getting smarter with our workouts.

We will cover four workouts, each with a similar structure to keep up the pace and keep you focused. If you are a beginner, you can slowly ramp these up so it's not too big a shock to your body. Taking guidance from your target body plan in the Goal Body Matrix, start with the Main Level workout as indicated. You might find that this is enough to attain your goal (as it did for me), or if you want faster results or you want to do more, you can move up to the Advanced Level workouts.

Finding the time

We all know the challenge of finding time to work out, so having short workouts gives you more flexibility to find a way to fit it in. Maybe it can be at the start of the day at home when you wake up. Maybe during lunch with friends or if you have a gym at work, or right when you get home.

You could even get off from your bus or train a stop earlier and then jog home! There are so many ways to fit workouts into your day. All it takes is a little creativity!

HIIT Style

To keep up the pace, we'll be using a fairly similar style of workout. High Intensity Interval Training, or HIIT for short, has become very popular in recent years, and for good reason:

- Workouts are short – around 20 minutes for most sessions
- It's more effective than long endurance training sessions[17]
- It's better than endurance training at burning fat[18]
- It increases resting metabolic rate for a full 24 hours after your workout, helping you to burn more fat[19]

This means you do a short workout that burns more body fat for longer than regular exercise. The proof is there, so all we need to do is use it and we can obtain lean and healthy bodies with much less effort and time than before.

What exactly is it?

HIIT has a simple format that comprises of a 'Work' interval and a 'Rest' interval. Each interval is timed to keep the pace and your heart rate up. Research has shown that a 2:1 Work to Rest ratio is best. The idea is to really get your heart rate up in the Work intervals so that you get very close to your maximum oxygen consumption rate, called 'VO2max', then allowing a quick recovery interval before getting back into it.

Calculating your VO2max involves some complicated maths, but essentially: during the workout, you have to really push it – your heart should be racing, you should be breathing heavily, you should be sweating. As a simple measure, you should not be able to have a conversation while you are working out since your body needs every breath just to keep you going.

The traditional form of HIIT is more a cardiovascular workout, where something like running or cycling is your main exercise for the whole workout. Though, we can use these same principles to construct more muscle toning workouts, so you build strength as well. We'll start with Pure HIIT workouts, which are more traditional cardiovascular style workouts. As we go through Body HIIT, Lean HIIT and Heavy HIIT, our workouts will become increasingly more strength-focused with less cardio.

What about Tabata?

Some of you may be familiar with the Tabata protocol, which is a format of exercise where you only do 4 minutes at super high intensity. So if that's even shorter than the HIIT exercises, why don't I include it here?

The reason is that when you reach that level of intensity, you become far more likely to injure yourself and dramatically set back your progress. If you do wish to try it, I suggest you do so with a qualified trainer to help you perform all the exercises with proper form and intensity.

Essentially what we are tuning through these different workouts is your endurance muscles versus your strength muscles. Endurance muscles are smaller and give you a slimmer look, while strength muscles give you power and muscles become more defined. Bodybuilders focus almost purely on strength muscles, while marathon runners focus on endurance muscles. Imagining the two, you can see how the different types of muscles result in different body types. This is why it's so important for you to be clear about the body you want to develop – so you can do the right exercises to achieve it!

Workout format

The workouts themselves last about 15 to 25 minutes. This makes it a great alternative to long cardio sessions and allows you to fit exercise into your schedule even if you are really busy. You can do them without any special equipment, so you can do your full workout at home or in the hotel room if you are travelling!

The workout follows a simple Work and Rest interval format. Depending on the program, you can use the following timing:

- 30 seconds Work, 15 seconds Rest
- 40 seconds Work, 20 seconds Rest

As you can see, the workouts are very fast paced. After 20 minutes you should be feeling wiped out. To help keep up the pace and keep track during the workout, a good HIIT timer application on your phone is almost a necessity since it will save you from having to keep an eye on a clock. If you look in your app store (iTunes, Google Play, etc.), just search for "interval timer" and you'll get a bunch of free options to try out.

Incorporating weights

Using weights is really important as the resistance gives your muscles a reason to get stronger. Higher muscle mass gives your body more shape, which is what you need to get that lean look. If you have not used weights before, don't worry – it is really easy! Like before, this plan has photos for each exercise so that you can see exactly how it is done.

You may have heard people in the gym talk about 'sets' and 'reps', but what do these two terms mean?

- **Repetition (rep)** – One rep is when you do one exercise from start to finish. For example, if you are doing a squat, starting at the top, squatting to the floor, and standing up again is one repetition
- **Set** – A set is a number of repetitions performed right after each other until you have a break. For example, you might do 10 reps of squats as one set and have a break. In a workout, you might do four sets of squats for 10 reps each, meaning in total you are doing 40 squats

Sets and reps are important as how you use them changes how your workouts affect your muscles. For example:

- If you do heavy weights, you can only do a few reps per set. This exercises your strength muscles (fast-contractile speed and are therefore suited to short fast bursts of power) which grow more and have a smaller effect on your cardiovascular health. This is why it is better for building an athletic body
- If you do lighter weights, you can do more reps. This exercises your endurance muscles (slow-contractile speed and are therefore suited to a steady pace for a longer duration) which grow less and are better for cardiovascular health. This is why it is better for developing a slimmer body

Knowing this, you can use the same exercise format to tailor the workout to your goals. To get a lean body, you need to use lighter weights. To get an athletic body, you need to use heavier weights. Simple!

Focus on form!

If you are new to working out, or even if you've been doing it a while, here is something important to remember – ***always focus on form***! Doing exercises with proper form is incredibly important to avoid injury and also make sure you are targeting the right muscles. Have a close look at the photos provided with each of the exercises, and never sacrifice form to complete an exercise. If you can't do an exercise with proper form anymore, take a rest and then start again. This will help you avoid injuries and still get good results!

4.1 Pure HIIT

The original form of HIIT that most research was conducted on was simple, one exercise sessions with alternating intensity. This would often be a stationary bicycle or treadmill. Because this is the original HIIT, we'll call these workouts "Pure HIIT". They are more cardiovascular in nature, meaning they work your heart, lungs and endurance muscles more than they work your strength muscles. This makes it a great workout if you are looking for a slim body type. It's also great to add in to other workouts if you want an extra fat burning boost.

Remember *– you have to do the right kind of exercise to get the body you want. Follow the guidance in the Goal Body Matrix to find the right workout for you!*

If you are looking for a simple but effective cardio workout, try the exercises below. These are single exercises you can use to vary the intensity over 20 minutes (or less) using different types of equipment:

- Stationery bike
- Treadmill
- Rowing machine
- Skipping rope
- Shoes
    - Go for a run
    - Or if you are stuck indoors, alternate between High Knees and jogging in place

Pick your preferred equipment and go for it! If you have access to more than one of the above, you can cycle through them each week to give yourself some variety.

The workout formula is super simple:

1. *Do a quick 1 minute warmup – slow pace of whatever exercise you're about to do*
2. *Set your interval timer to 30 seconds 'Work' and 15 seconds 'Rest' for 26 rounds (total of 20 minutes), or 20 rounds (total of 15 minutes) for a faster workout.*
3. *Get started and sprint as hard as you can for 30 seconds, then slow down for 15 seconds while you rest – repeat for all 26 rounds*
4. *Finish with a bit of stretching to cool down –* ***DONE!***

4.2 Body HIIT

Beyond the Pure HIIT exercises, doing a whole-body workout will build more strength and give you a toned body. Here you want to do exercises that not only get your heart rate up, but also exercise muscles all over your body to achieve a balanced and lean figure.

Each workout is set up as a circuit - you do an exercise for 40 seconds, rest for 20, then move on to the next exercise until you've reached the last exercise, and then start over again. This is going to keep you focused and your body challenged along the way.

Equipment needed

For the most part you will be doing body-weight exercises (hence "Body HIIT"!), so you only need a few dumbbells to get a full body workout. If you are just starting out, I'd recommend you get:

- 2x 1kg (2.5lb) dumbbells
- 2x 2kg (5lb) dumbbells

If you find these weights really easy during the workouts, then get 2x 4kg (10lb) dumbbells and step it up!

Body HIIT Workout Plan

The Body HIIT plan has five main workouts you can cycle through in the week. Each workout consists of five exercises that you cycle through in a circuit. You can do more, or fewer days of these, depending on what you have time for and how fast you want to achieve your goals. I'd recommend to try and fit in all five workouts in a week - it's only about 20 minutes each, so you don't need much time at all! If you want to do more than five days a week, then you can repeat workouts as you like.

If you are getting to a more advanced level and want a bigger challenge, try out the two Advanced Workouts included.

The workout formula goes like this:

1. *Do a quick 1 minute warmup – 20 seconds walking in place, 20 seconds jog in place, 20 seconds jumping jacks*

2. *Set your interval timer to 40 seconds 'Work' and 20 seconds 'Rest' for 20 rounds (total of 20 minutes)*

3. *Get started and do each exercise for 40 seconds, then rest for 20 seconds. Move on to the next exercise for the next 40 seconds, and start back at the beginning when you've done all of them, for a total of 20 rounds.*

4. *Finish with a bit of stretching to cool down – **DONE!***

BODY HIIT WORKOUT

DAY 1

Circuit training! Do 40 seconds of each exercise, rest for 20 seconds, then do the next exercise for a total of 20 rounds until you have done each exercise 4 times.

Equipment	Sturdy chair
Intervals	Work - 40 seconds Rest - 20 seconds
Rounds	20 rounds = 20 minutes in total

1 Bicycle Abs

- Lie on your back with your hands behind your head
- Lift up both legs and bring your left knee to your right elbow, contracting your abs
- Swap sides and keep going for the duration of the round

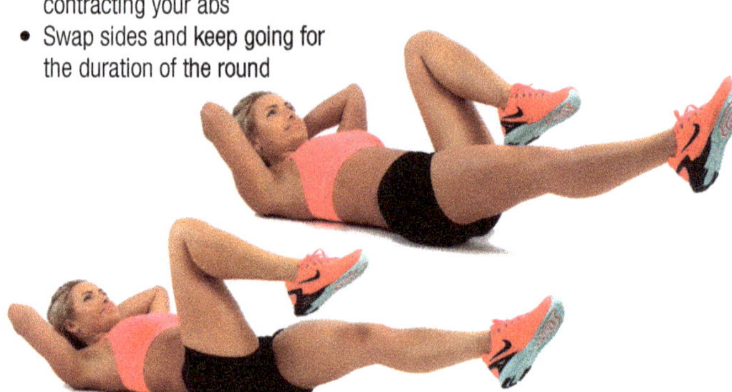

2 Side Lunge Jumps

- Squat halfway down on one leg, hand touching the ground
- Point your other leg straight and off to the side
- Power up into a jump while bringing the outer leg in and pointing the inner leg out
- Jump while alternating between legs

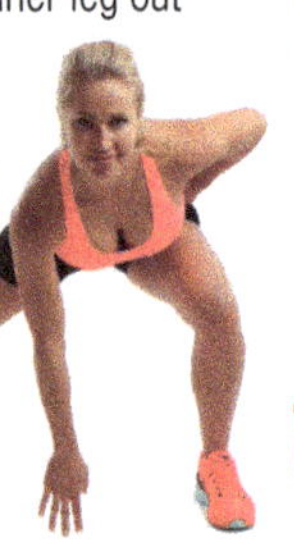

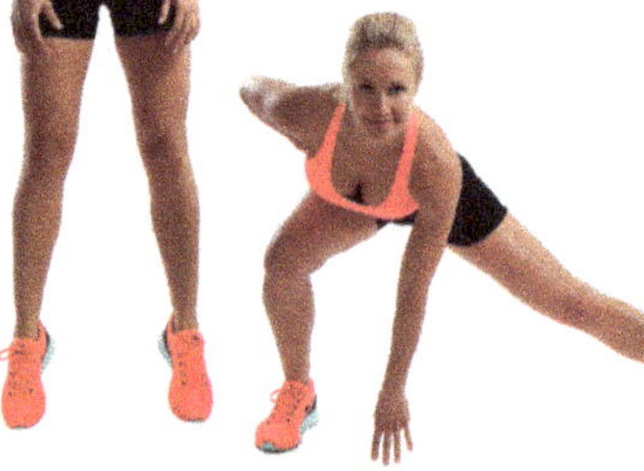

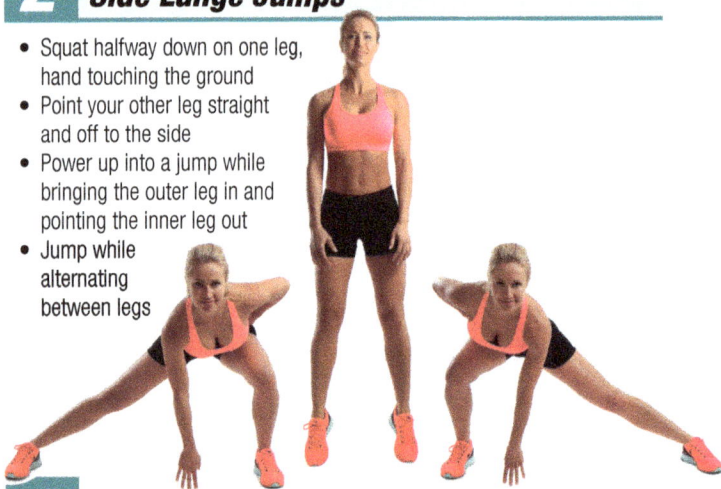

3 Pushup Onto Chair

- Go into a pushup position with your hands resting on the edge of a chair
- Keep your back and legs straight and lower until your chest touches the bench
- Push back up to the starting position

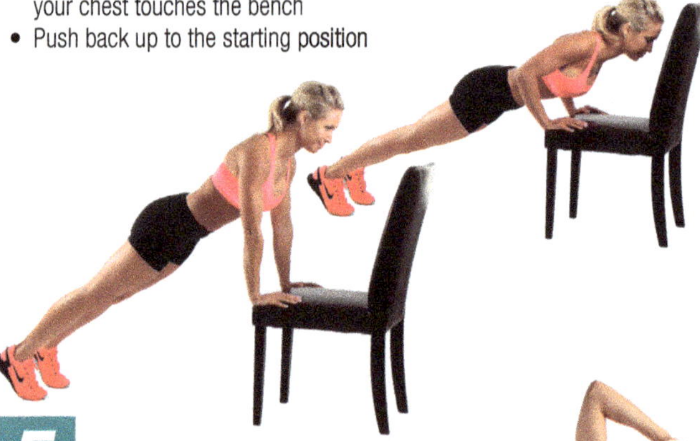

4 Scissor Kicks

- Lie on your back with your hands behind your head
- Lift both legs off the ground, then bring one leg up 90 degrees to your body
- Swap legs, keeping both legs straight throughout
- Keep your head off the ground by contracting your abs all the way

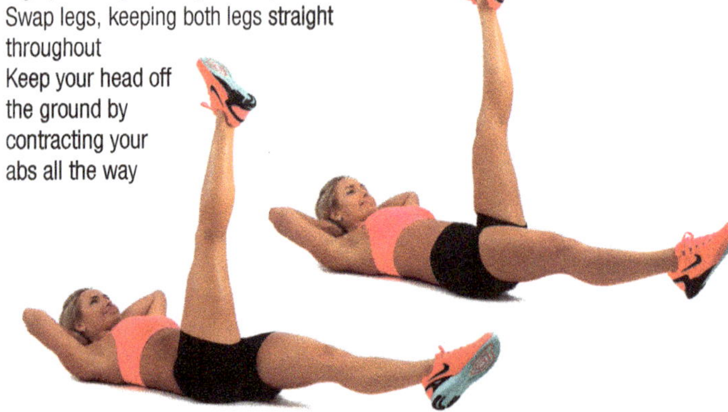

5 Squat Knee-ups

- Start standing while holding your arms behind your head
- Squat down, keep the weight on your heels
- Push up from your heel while bringing one knee up to your elbow on the other side
- Return your foot to the ground and repeat, alternating between legs

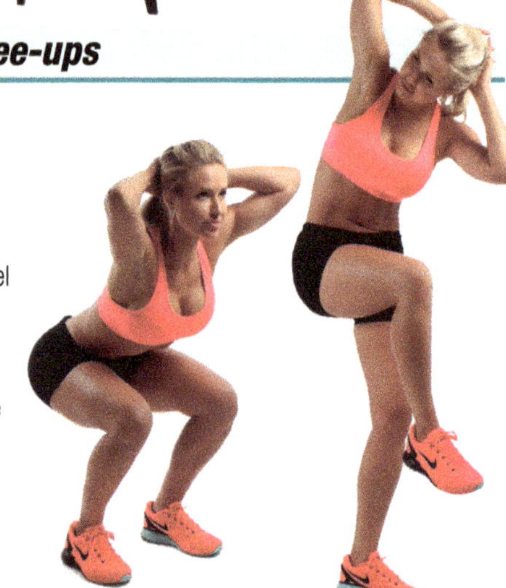

FAST WARMUP: 20 secs walk in place, 20 secs jog in place, 20 secs jumping jacks

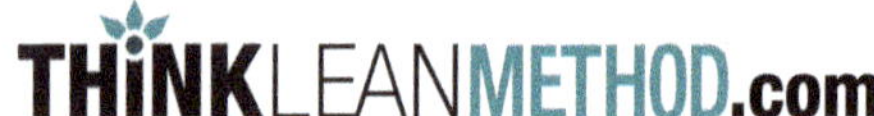

BODY HIIT WORKOUT

DAY 2

Circuit training! Do 40 seconds of each exercise, rest for 20 seconds, then do the next exercise for a total of 20 rounds until you have done each exercise 4 times.

Equipment Dumbbells

Intervals Work - 40 seconds
Rest - 20 seconds

Rounds 20 rounds = 20 minutes in total

1 Mountain Climbers

- Start in a sprinting position
- Keeping hands on the ground, bring one knee into your chest while kicking the other leg back
- Keep going by swapping legs in a running motion

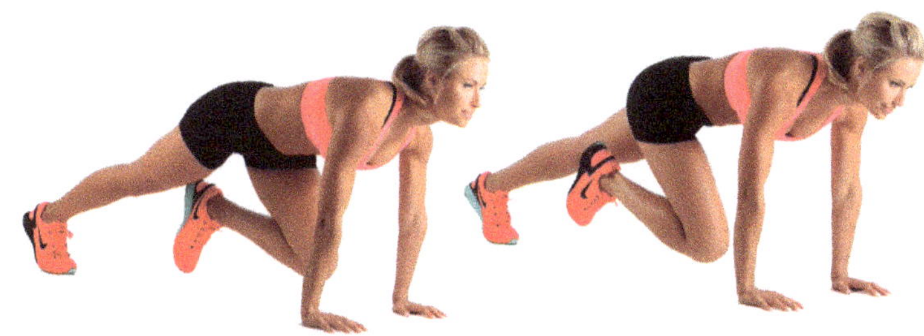

2 Burpees

- Start by doing a normal pushup
- As you push up, kick in your legs and go into a squat position
- From there, power into a jump with your arms reaching to the sky
- Land back in a squat position and go back into a pushup

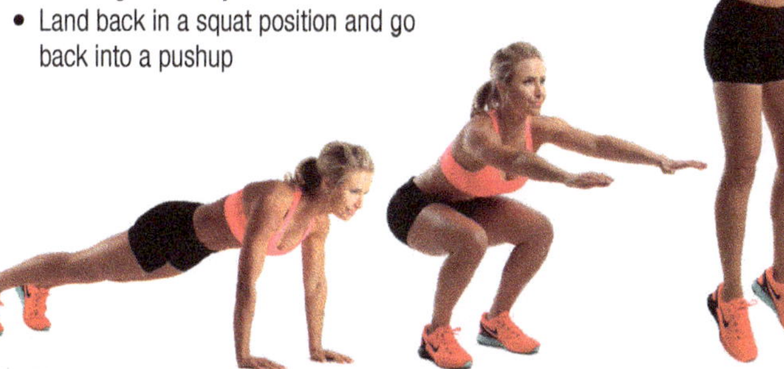

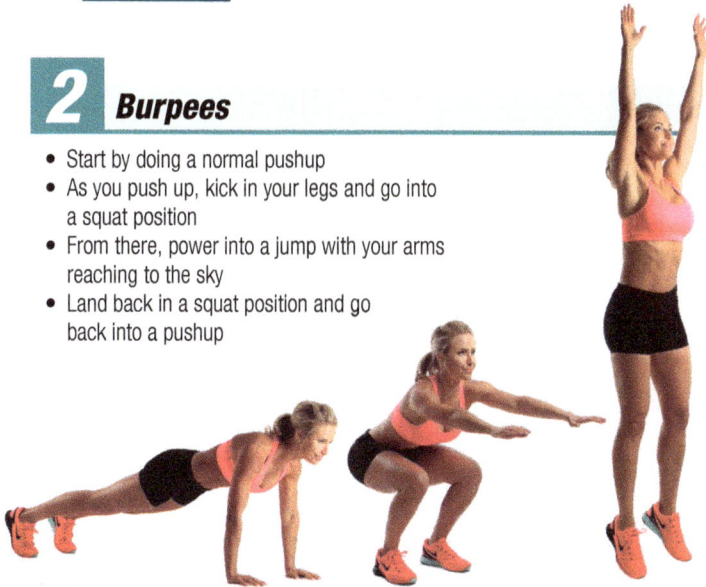

3 Curl And Press

- Start with dumbbells hanging by your waist with thumbs pointing outwards
- Lift the weights by curling your biceps
- From there extend your arms upwards to complete the press
- Lower the weights back to your shoulders
- Then lower back down to your waist

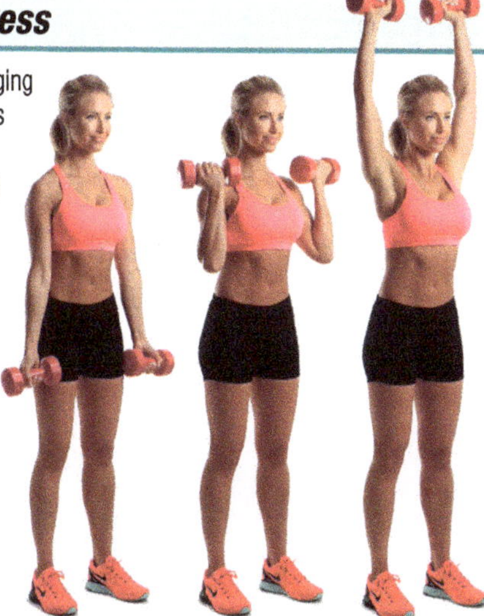

4 Glute Kickbacks

- Start on all fours, holding your back straight
- Lift one leg upwards as far as you can go, squeezing your glutes
- Lower the leg and swap with the other leg

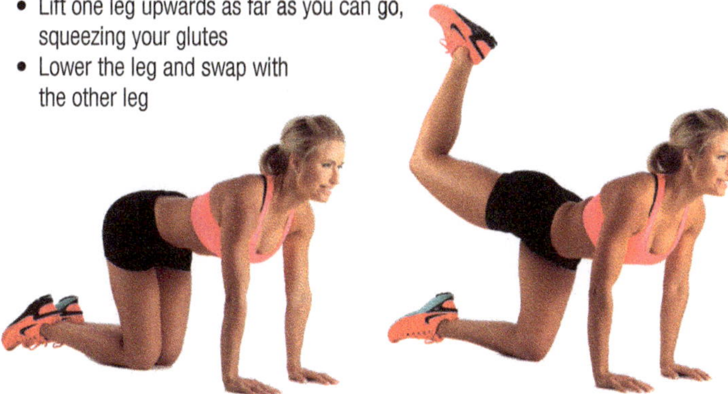

5 Leg Lift Pushups

- Start in a pushup position, holding your back straight
- Lift one leg upwards behind you
- Do a pushup holding your leg up, then swap legs

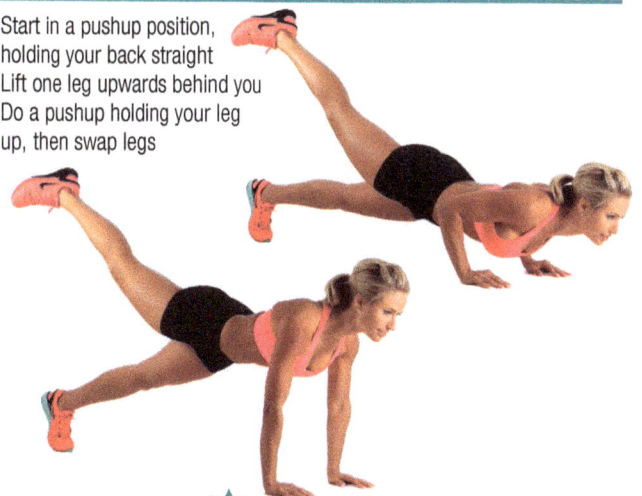

FAST WARMUP: 20 secs walk in place, 20 secs jog in place, 20 secs jumping jacks

BODY HIIT WORKOUT

DAY 3

Circuit training! Do 40 seconds of each exercise, rest for 20 seconds, then do the next exercise for a total of 20 rounds until you have done each exercise 4 times.

Equipment	Workout bench or chair + Dumbbells
Intervals	Work - 40 seconds Rest - 20 seconds
Rounds	20 rounds = 20 minutes in total

1 *Walking Lunges*

- Start in a lunge position
- Keep legs bent at 90 degree angles
- Push forward from your back leg to go into a standing position
- Return to the lunge position and repeat so that you continually move forward

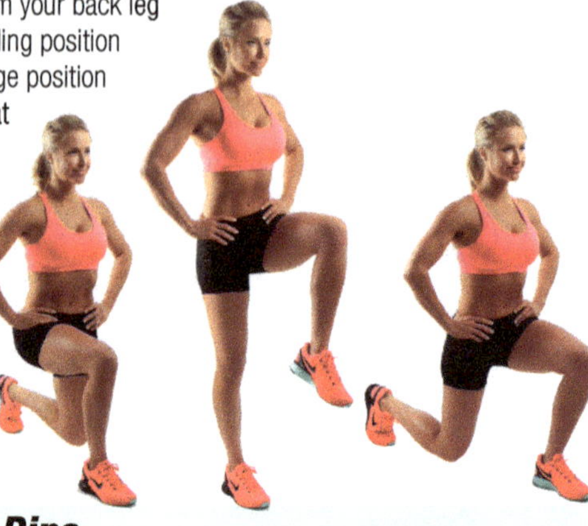

2 *V-sit*

- Keeping both your legs and back straight, sit in a V position while balancing on your buttocks
- Hold the position for the duration of the set

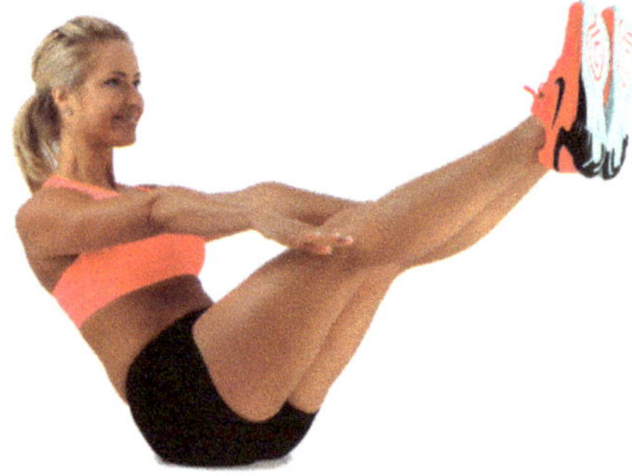

3 *Bench Dips*

- Legs extended away from the bench and bent at the waist, put your hands on a bench behind your back
- Bend your elbows and lower down until your elbows are about shoulder-height
- Push back up to the starting position

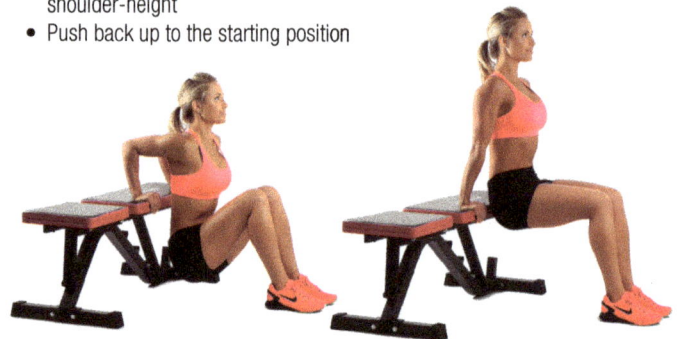

4 *Dumbbell Bent Over Rows*

- Hold a dumbbell in each hand and bend over at the waist
- Pull up the dumbbells, keeping your elbows close to your sides
- Drop the weights back in front of you

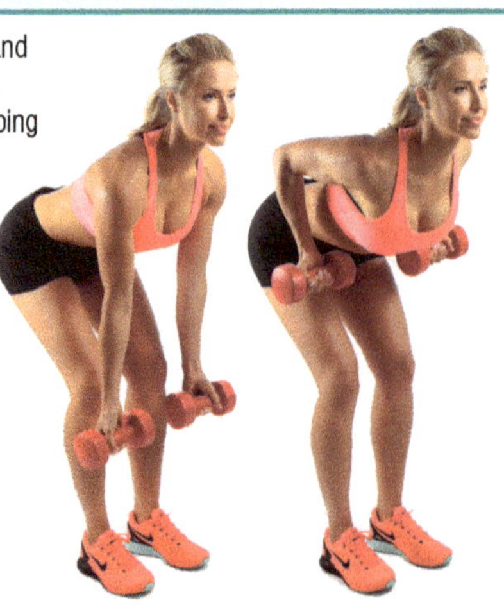

5 *Glute Kickbacks*

- Start on all fours, holding your back straight
- Lift one leg upwards as far as you can go, squeezing your glutes
- Lower the leg and swap with the other leg

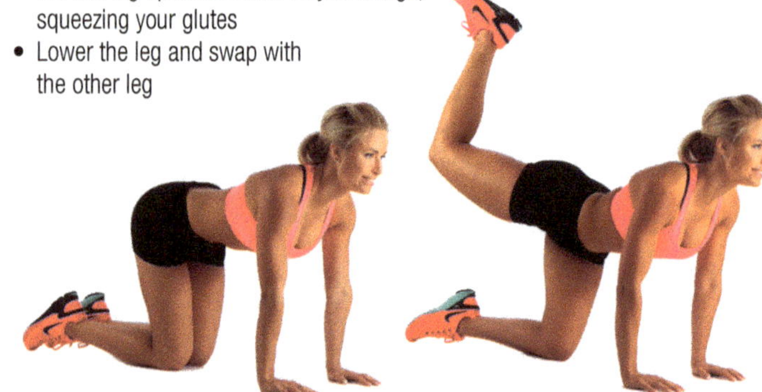

FAST WARMUP: 20 secs walk in place, 20 secs jog in place, 20 secs jumping jacks

BODY HIIT WORKOUT

DAY 4

Circuit training! Do 40 seconds of each exercise, rest for 20 seconds, then do the next exercise for a total of 20 rounds until you have done each exercise 4 times.

Equipment Dumbbells

Intervals Work - 40 seconds
Rest - 20 seconds

Rounds 20 rounds = 20 minutes in total

1 *Leg Lift Pushups*

- Start in a pushup position, holding your back straight
- Lift one leg upwards behind you
- Do a pushup holding your leg up, then swap legs

2 *Alternating Lunges*

- Start in the standing position
- Drop forward into a lunge with your left leg forward, keeping legs bent at 90 degree angles
- Push back with your left leg into the starting position
- Repeat with your right leg

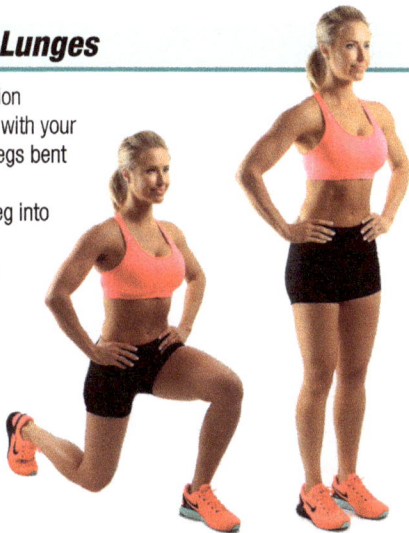

3 *Dumbbell Reverse Flyes*

- Hold dumbbells in each hand and bend over at the waist, keeping your back straight
- Keep your arms slightly bent and stiff, and swing them out to the sides, squeezing your shoulder blades
- Return to the starting position in a slow and controlled motion

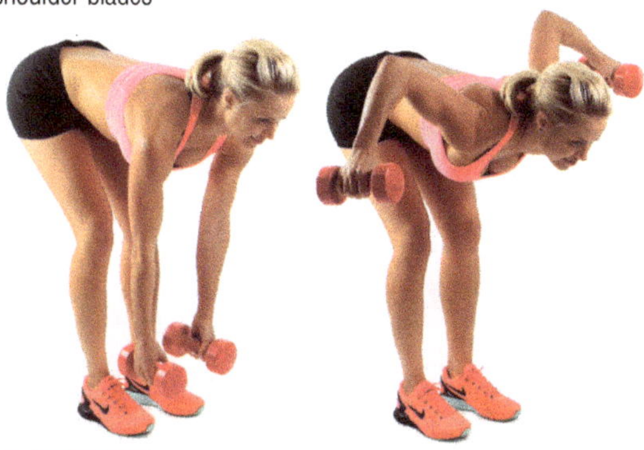

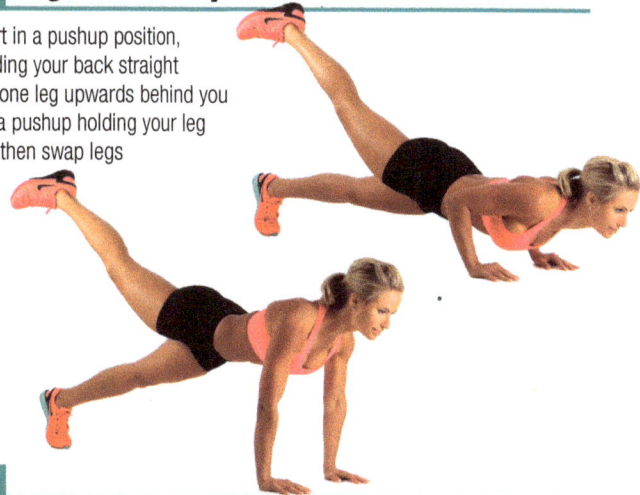

4 *Swings*

- Hold on to a dumbbell in front of you with both hands
- Squat down halfway so the dumbbell is between your legs – keep your back straight
- Power up from your buttocks and use momentum to swing the weight up to shoulder-height
- Swing back into a squat, keeping arms straight the whole time
- Keep momentum going for the entire set

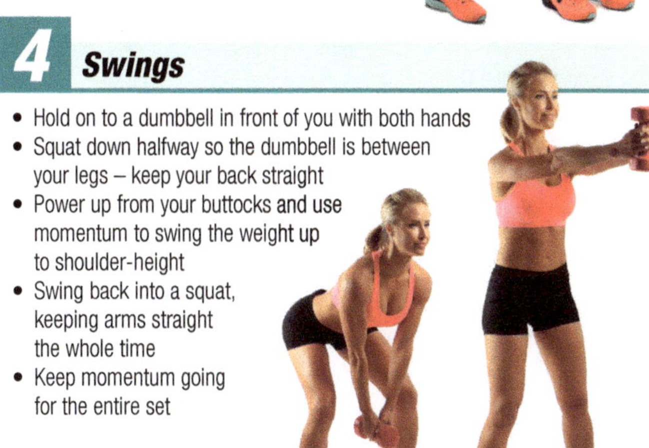

5 *Russian Twist*

- Start in a sit-up position, holding a weight with both hands in front of you
- Twist at your waist from side to side, while holding your arms stiff

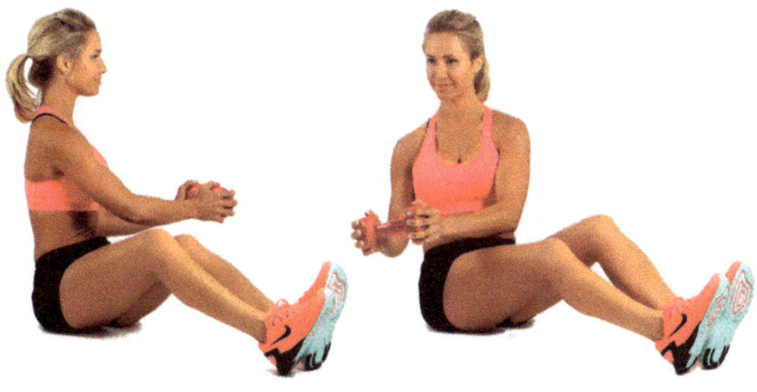

FAST WARMUP: 20 secs walk in place, 20 secs jog in place, 20 secs jumping jacks

BODY HIIT WORKOUT

DAY 5

Circuit training! These 7 exercises total 10 rounds (some of them have to be repeated for the other side of your body). Do the circuit twice for a total of 20 minutes!

Equipment Dumbbells

Intervals Work - 40 seconds
Rest - 20 seconds

Rounds 20 rounds = 20 minutes in total

1 Lunge Kick-ups

- Start in a lunge position with the left leg behind you and right arm held out in front
- Power up from your back leg and kick across your body so your foot touches your outstretched hand
- Return your leg back behind you to the starting position
- Do a set on one leg then another set on the other leg

40 seconds with your left leg, rest, then 40 seconds with your right leg

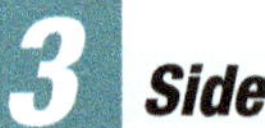

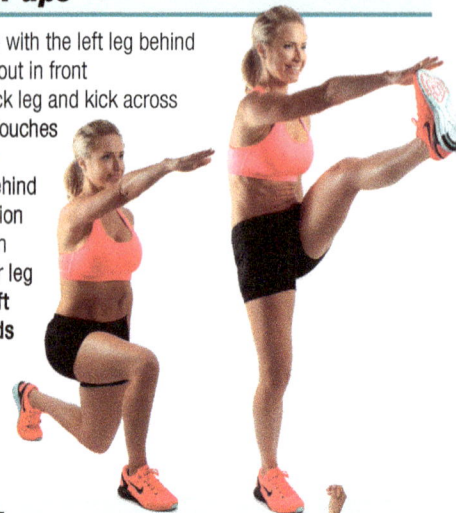

2 Pushups

- Put your hands on the floor about shoulder-width apart, keeping both your back and legs straight
- Slowly lower down until your chest touches the ground
- For an easier version, pivot on your knees instead of feet

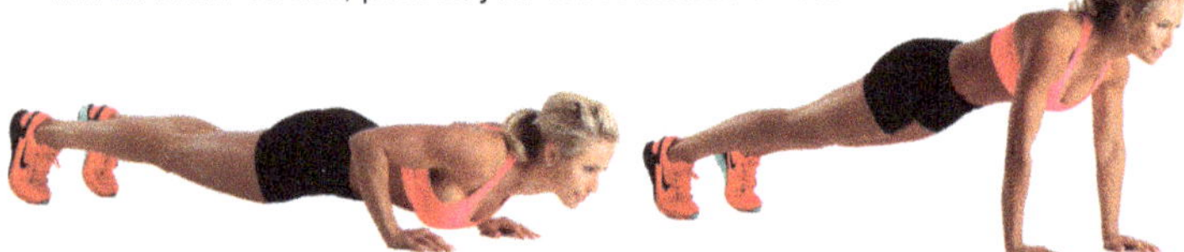

3 Side Plank

- Hold your body straight while extending one arm with your hand on the floor
- Maintain the position for the duration of the set, then swap sides

40 seconds on your left side, rest, then 40 seconds on the right side

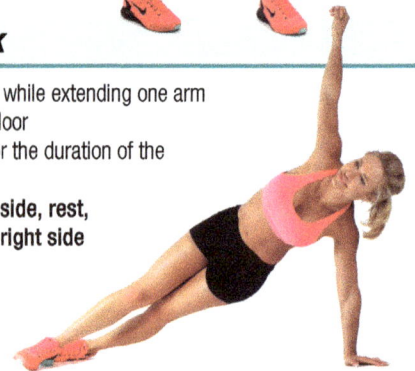

4 Pulse Squats

- Keeping your back straight and weight on your heels, squat down until your thighs are parallel to the floor
- Lift up about 15 cm (7 inches) and drop back down to the starting position, continuing in a pulsing motion for the duration of the set

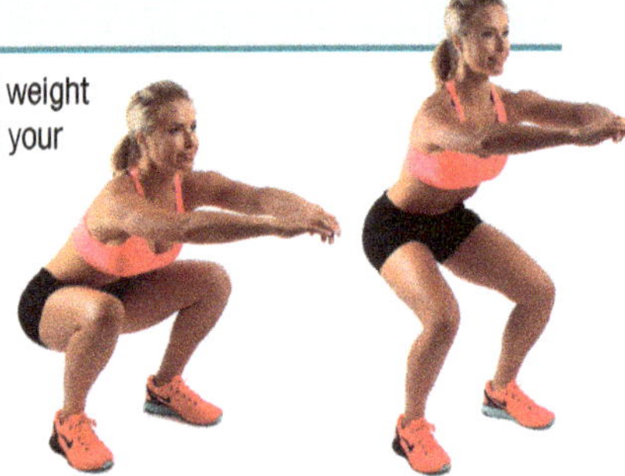

5 Dumbbell Curl and Press

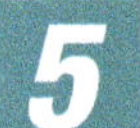

- Start with dumbbells hanging by your waist with thumbs pointing outwards
- Lift the weights by curling your biceps
- From there extend your arms upwards to complete the press
- Lower the weights back to your shoulders
- Then lower back down to your waist

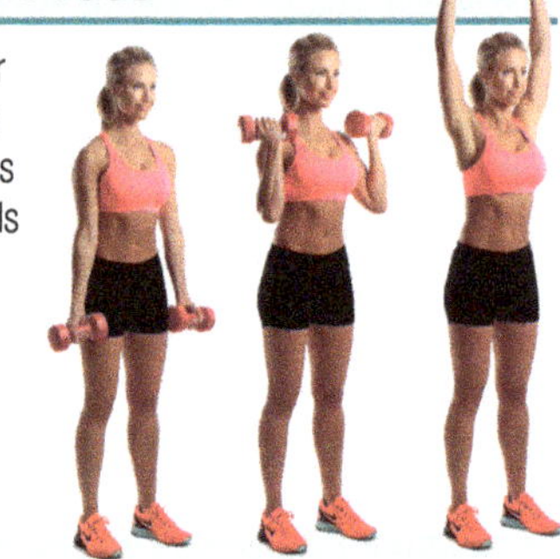

6 Forwards Backwards Lunge

- Start in the standing position
- Drop forward into a lunge with your left leg forward, legs bent at 90 degree angles
- Push back with your left leg and go directly into a backwards lunge position with your left leg now behind you
- Continue going back and forward, do another set with your right leg

40 seconds with your left leg, rest, then 40 seconds with your right leg

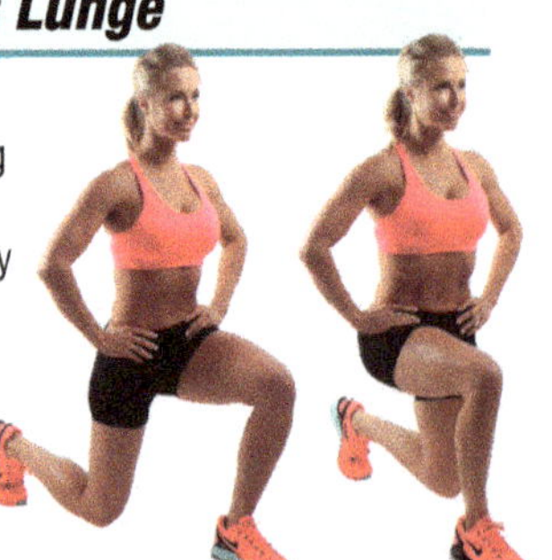

7 Flutter Kicks

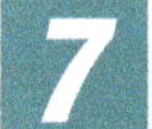

- Lying on your back on the floor with arms by your side, lift up both legs while keeping them straight
- Move one foot down slightly and the other up at the same time
- In quick succession, alternate your legs

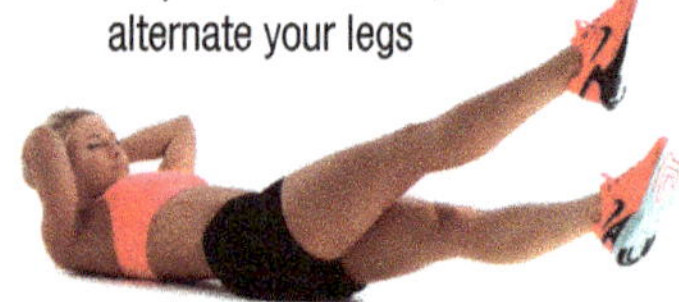

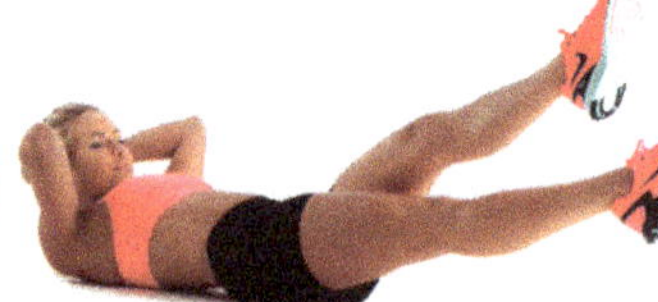

FAST WARMUP: 20 secs walk in place, 20 secs jog in place, 20 secs jumping jacks

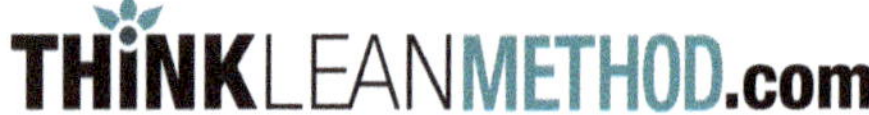

ADVANCED HIIT WORKOUT

ADV 1

Circuit training! Do 40 seconds of each exercise, rest for 20 seconds, then do the next exercise for a total of 20 rounds until you have done each exercise 4 times.

Equipment Workout bench, bed or sofa

Intervals Work - 40 seconds
Rest - 20 seconds

Rounds 20 rounds = 20 minutes in total

1 Hip Thrust

- Rest your shoulders on a bench (a bed or sofa can work), arms stretched out and hold on to stabilise yourself
- Keep one foot on the ground with knee bent at 90 degrees
- Hold the other leg in the air
- Drop down by bending at your waist and push back up until your body is parallel to the ground
- Do 20 reps and swap sides

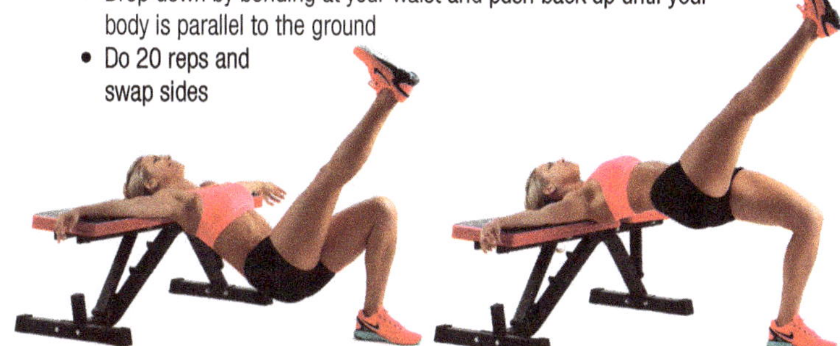

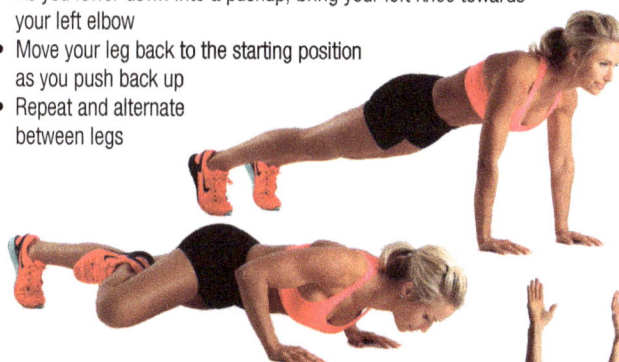

2 High Knees Jog

- Jog in place, each time driving up your knee as high as you can
- Keep up the pace for the full duration of the round
- Keep your core tight and chest up

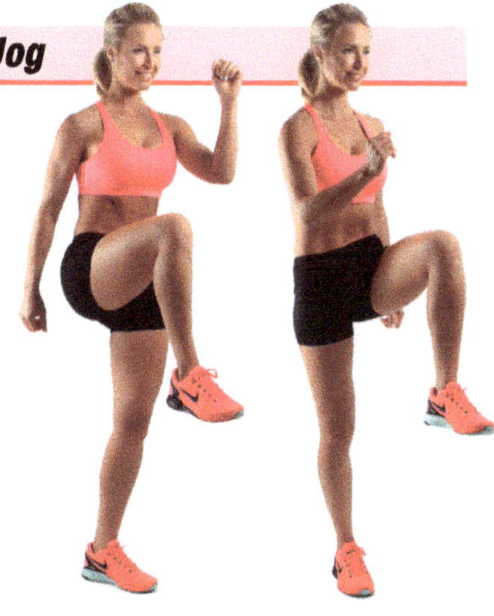

3 Knee To Elbow Pushups

- Start in a pushup position with your hands about shoulder-width apart
- As you lower down into a pushup, bring your left knee towards your left elbow
- Move your leg back to the starting position as you push back up
- Repeat and alternate between legs

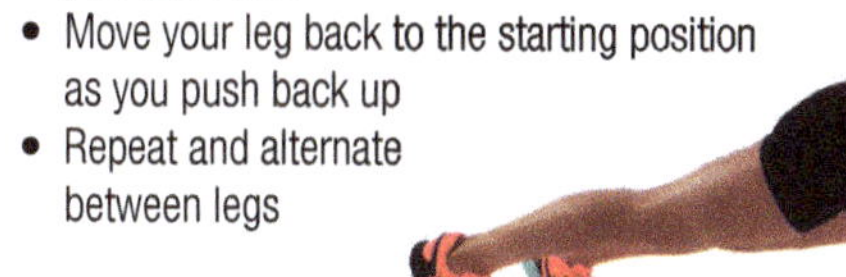

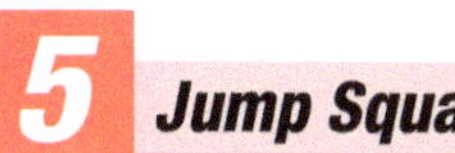

4 Windshield Wipers

- Lie on the floor with your arms outstretched and both legs in the air at 90 degrees to your body
- Keeping your legs straight, lower them to the right until your right leg touches the ground
- Bring them back up and repeat on the other side

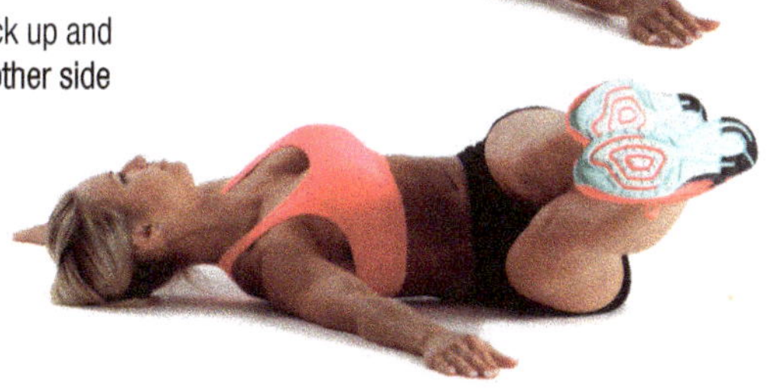

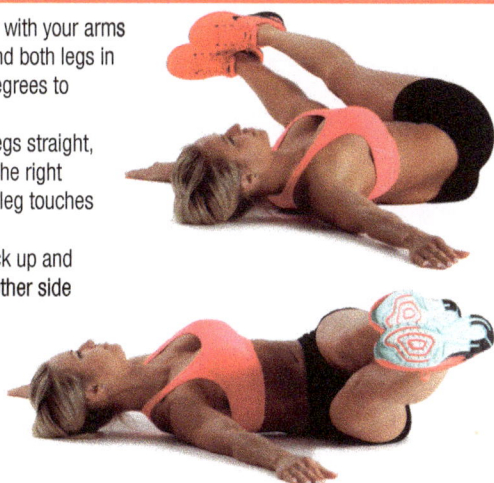

5 Jump Squat

- Start with your arms out in front of you
- Squat down, keep the weight on your heels
- Power up from your heels into a jump and land again in a squat

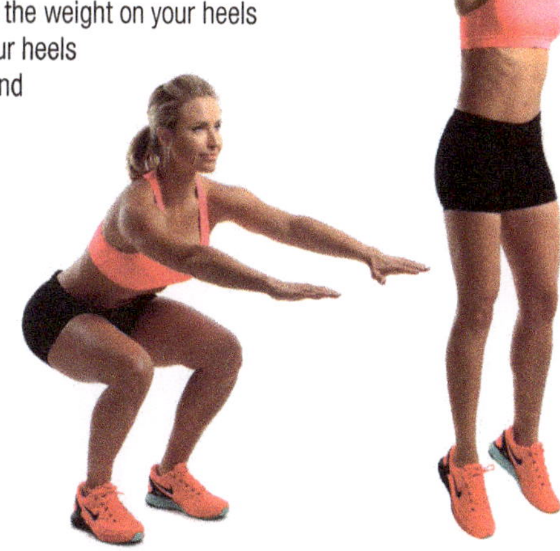

FAST WARMUP: 20 secs walk in place, 20 secs jog in place, 20 secs jumping jacks

ADVANCED HIIT WORKOUT

ADV 2

Circuit training! Do 40 seconds of each exercise, rest for 20 seconds, then do the next exercise for a total of 20 rounds until you have done each exercise 4 times.

Equipment	Dumbbells
Intervals	Work - 40 seconds Rest - 20 seconds
Rounds	20 rounds = 20 minutes in total

1 *Pistol Squats*

- Start by standing on one leg, other leg and arms pointed forwards
- While balancing, squat down on one leg until your thigh is parallel to the ground
- Push back up from your heel, keeping your back straight and core tight
- If you need help to balance, put one hand on the back of a chair, taking care not to pull yourself up with your hand

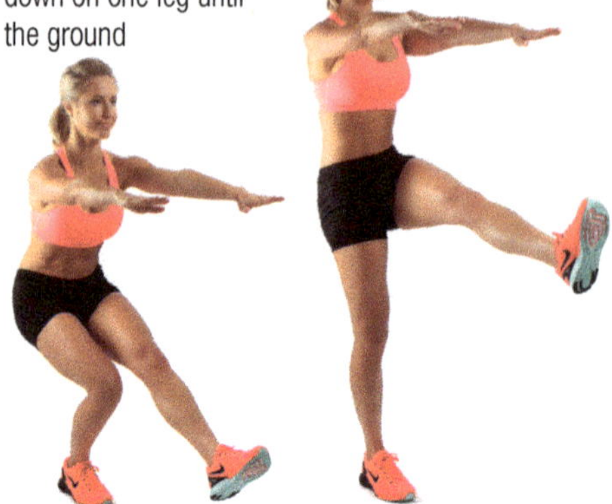

2 *Leg Lift Pushups*

- Start in a pushup position, holding your back straight
- Lift one leg upwards behind you
- Do a pushup holding your leg up, then swap legs

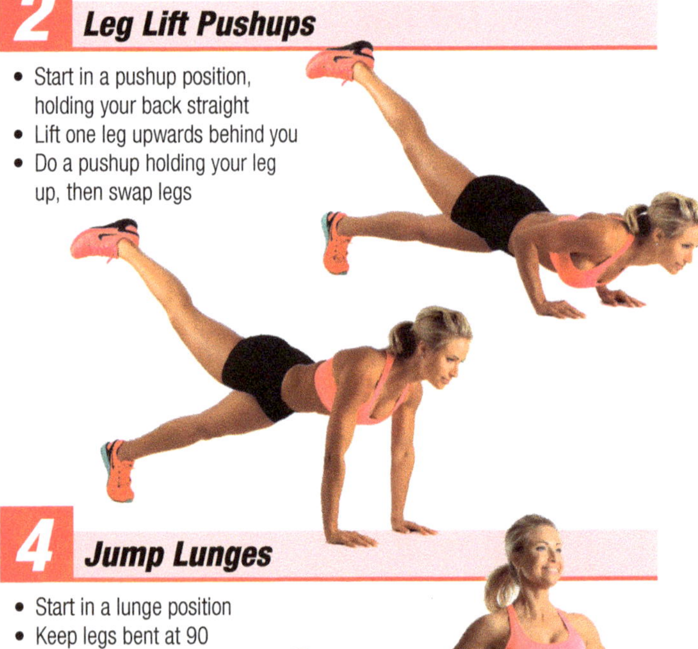

3 *V-sit*

- Keeping both your legs and back straight, sit in a V position while balancing on your buttocks
- Hold the position for the duration of the set

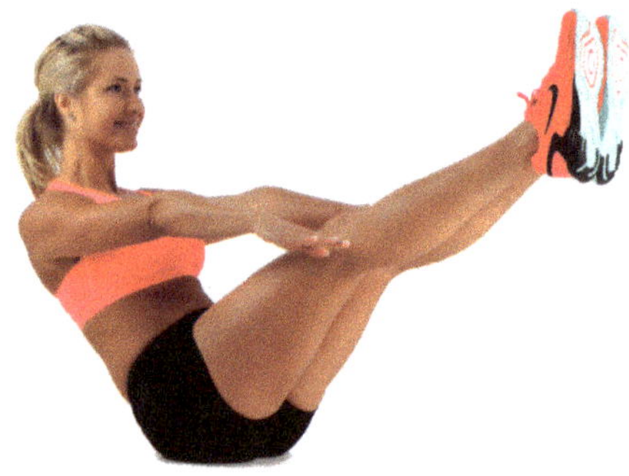

4 *Jump Lunges*

- Start in a lunge position
- Keep legs bent at 90 degree angles
- Power into a jump, swap legs in the air and land back in a lunge

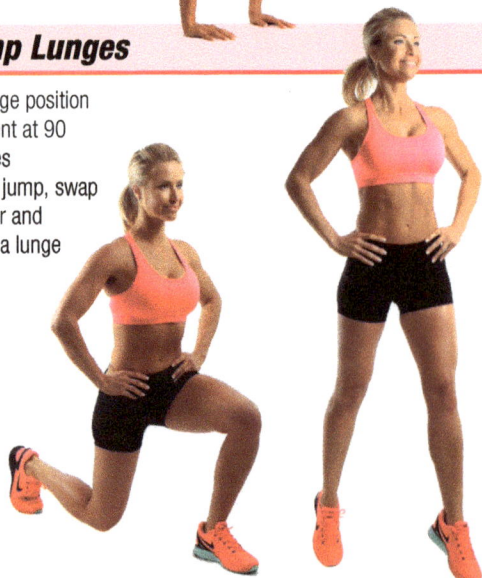

5 *Dumbbell Curl And Press*

- Start with dumbbells hanging by your waist with thumbs pointing outwards
- Lift the weights by curling your biceps
- From there extend your arms upwards to complete the press
- Lower the weights back to your shoulders
- Then lower back down to your waist

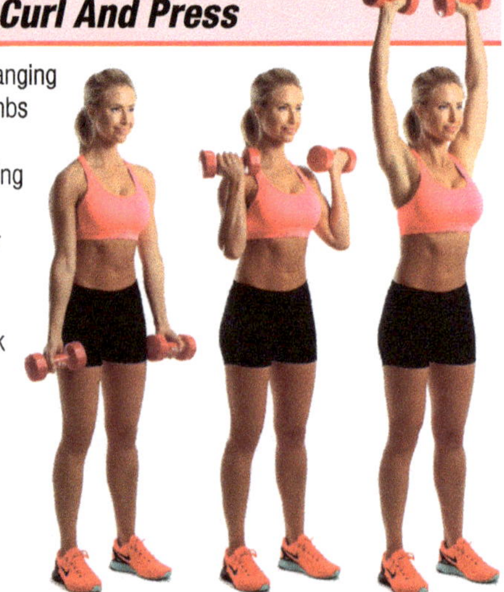

FAST WARMUP: 20 secs walk in place, 20 secs jog in place, 20 secs jumping jacks

4.3 Lean HIIT

For a more balanced full body workout, Lean HIIT steps it up to include more upper body elements. This is a fantastic plan for if you want to build an evenly strong and toned body. To do this, we are going to use weights more often.

These workouts go for 24 rounds each for a total of 24 minutes. Each workout is set up as a circuit - you do an exercise for 40 seconds, rest for 20, then move on to the next exercise until you've reached the last exercise, and then start over again. This is going to keep you focused and your body challenged along the way.

Equipment needed

The great thing about this workout is that with a little bit of equipment, you can do it all at home! An adjustable workout bench can come in handy, or you can just use the floor and a bed. You only need a few dumbbells to get a full body workout. If you are just starting out, I'd recommend you get:

- 2x 1kg dumbbells
- 2x 2kg dumbbells
- 2x 4kg dumbbells

If you find these weights really easy during the workouts, then get 2x 6kg dumbbells (or heavier) and step it up. If you feel like you are getting really strong, go for a set of adjustable dumbbells so that you can keep upping the weight without having to buy more dumbbells.

Lean HIIT Workout Plan

Unlike Body HIIT which is a full body workout each time, Lean HIIT focuses on specific muscle groups for each day. In this way, Lean HIIT has three workouts overall:

1. **Upper body** - Chest, back and shoulder muscles
2. **Lower body** - Quadriceps, hamstrings, calves and gluteus maximus
3. **Arms** - Biceps and triceps

If you want to do four workouts in a week, repeat workout 2 (lower body). You can also add in Pure HIIT workouts for additional fat burning.

To give you a uniquely effective mix, each workout consists of three types of exercises:

1. **Primary muscle movers** - These directly target the muscle group you are going after for that day. For these exercises, find a weight or level where you can do 20 reps for a set. Lower the weight if you can't reach 20, or increase the weight if you can do more than 20
2. **Cardio blasts** - These get your heart racing for added fat burning effect. Do these for the full 40 seconds interval
3. **Abdominals** - Each workout day includes an abdominal exercise to get your core tighter than ever before. Do these for the full 40 seconds interval

The workout formula goes like this:

1. *Do a quick 1 minute warmup – 20 seconds walking in place, 20 seconds jog in place, 20 seconds jumping jacks*

2. *Set your interval timer to 40 seconds 'Work' and 20 seconds 'Rest' for 24 rounds (total of 24 minutes)*

3. *Get started and do each of the exercises as indicated on the plans. Rest between each for 20 seconds and move on to the next exercise. Start back at the beginning when you've done all of them, for a total of 24 rounds*

4. *Finish with a bit of stretching to cool down – **DONE!***

LEAN HIIT UPPER BODY

DAY 1

Equipment Workout bench, or use the floor+ Dumbbells

Intervals Work - 40 seconds
Rest - 20 seconds

Rounds 24 rounds = 24 minutes in total

1 *Chest Press* - 20 reps

- Lie on a bench and hold dumbbells in each hand just above your chest, keeping elbows pointed down (do on the floor if you don't have a bench)
- Push the weights upwards, focusing on contracting your chest muscles
- Lower down to the starting position in a slow and controlled movement

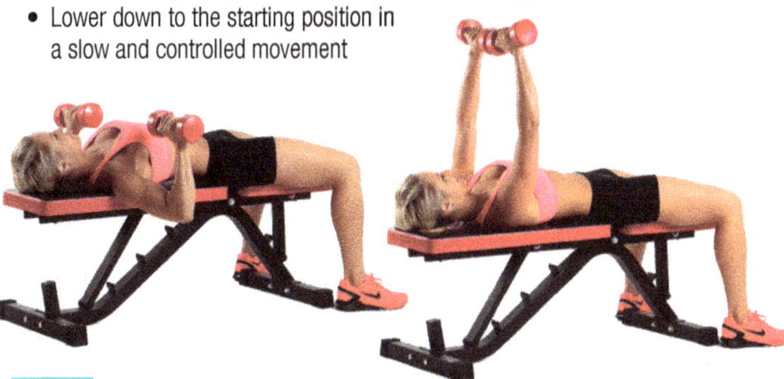

2 *Standing Shoulder Press* - 20 reps

- Start with dumbbells at shoulder height, thumbs facing backward
- Extend your arms upwards in a slow and controlled motion
- Slowly lower down to shoulder height and repeat

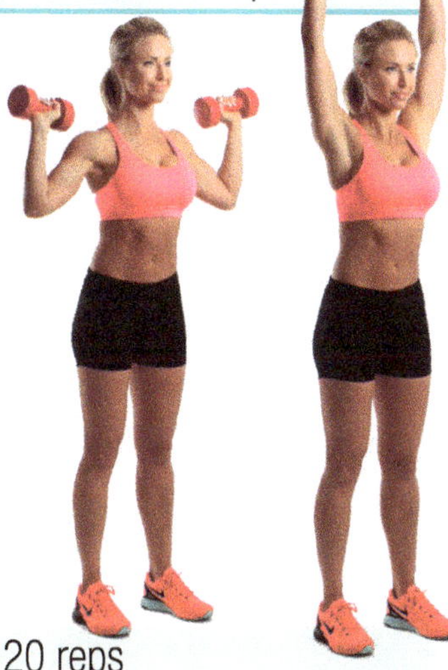

3 *Cardio Blast!* *Mountain Climbers* - 40 s

- Start in a sprinting position
- Keeping hands on the ground, bring one knee into your chest while kicking the other leg back
- Keep going by swapping legs in a running motion

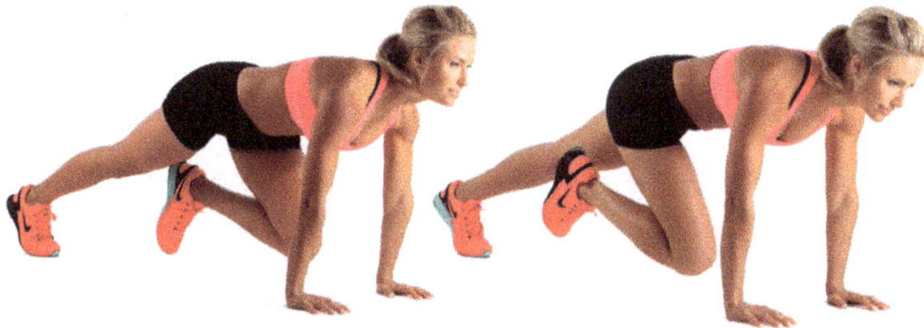

4 *Bent Over Rows* - 20 reps

- Hold a dumbbell in each hand and bend over at the waist
- Pull up the dumbbells, keeping your elbows close to your sides
- Drop the weights back in front of you

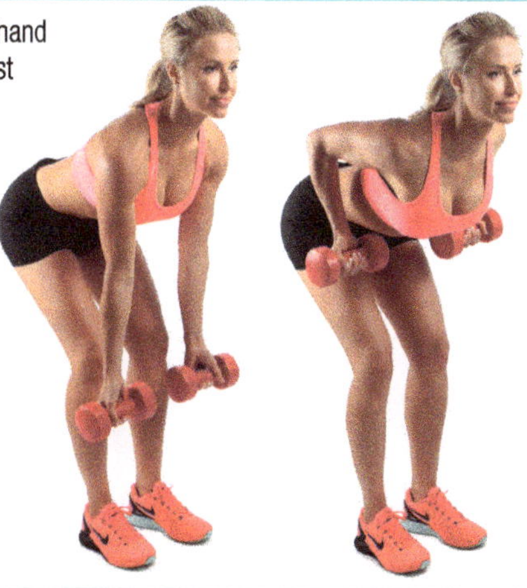

5 *Lateral Raises* - 20 reps

- In a standing position, hold dumbbells by each side
- Back of your hand facing outwards, keep your arms straight and lift up the weights outward to shoulder height
- Return down in a slow and controlled movement

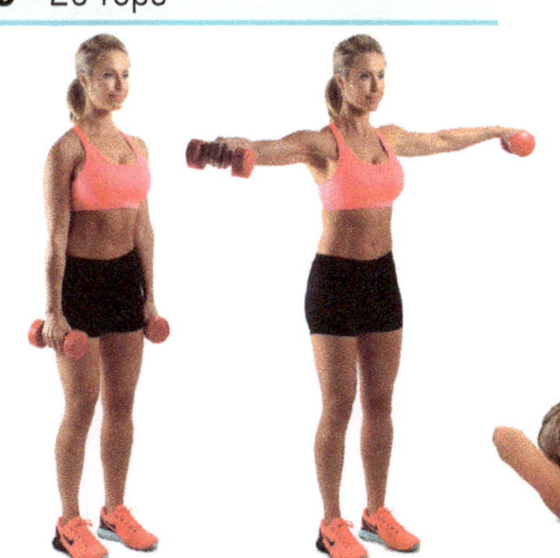

6 *Abs!* *Bicycle Abs* - 40 secs

- Lie on your back with your hands behind your head
- Lift up both legs and bring your left knee to your right elbow, contracting your abs
- Swap sides and keep going for the duration of the set

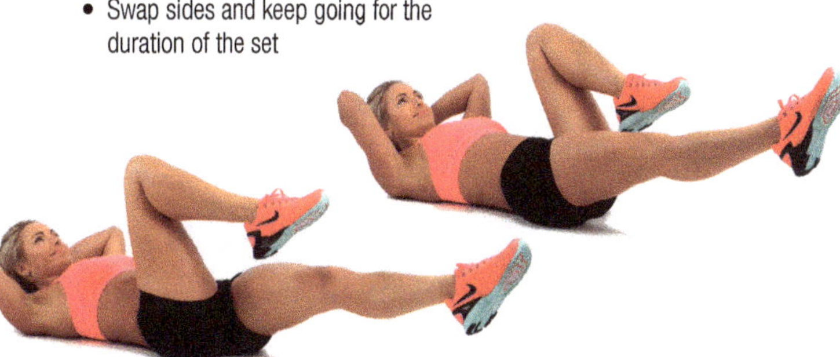

FAST WARMUP: 20 secs walk in place, 20 secs jog in place, 20 secs jumping jacks

LEAN HIIT LEGS & GLUTES DAY 2

Equipment Dumbbells

Intervals Work - 40 seconds
Rest - 20 seconds

Rounds 24 rounds = 24 minutes in total

1 *Goblet Squats* - 20 reps

- Take one dumbbell in both hands and hold it close to your chest
- Squat down until your thighs are at least parallel to the floor, keeping your back straight
- Return to a standing position
- If you have access to a squat rack, do normal squats with a barbell on your shoulders

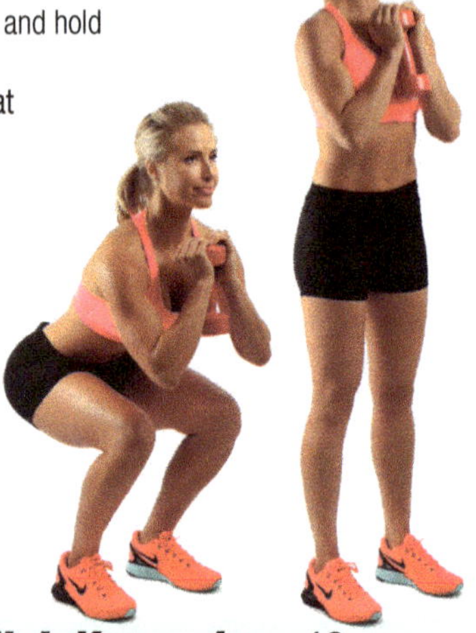

2 *Stiff Leg Deadlift* - 20 reps

- Start in a standing position, holding dumbbells in each hand
- Keeping your back straight, bend over from the waist until you feel a stretch in the back of your legs
- Return to the starting position in a slow and controlled movement
- Do with a barbell if you have access to one

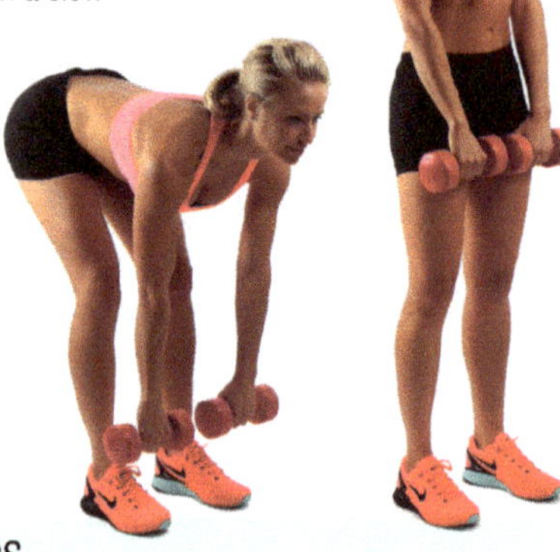

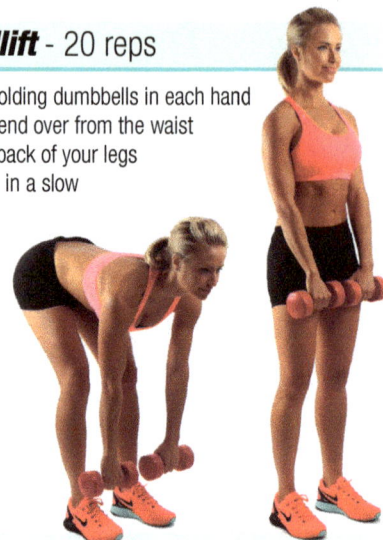

3 *Cardio Blast!* *High Knees Jog* - 40 secs

- Jog in place, each time driving up your knee as high as you can
- Keep up the pace for the full duration of the round
- Keep your core tight and chest up

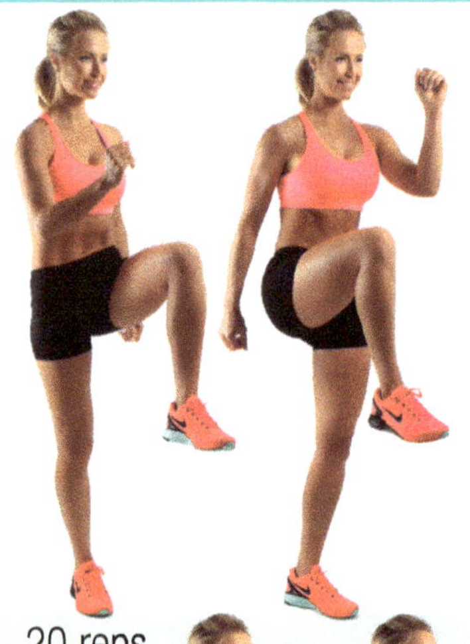

4 *Swings* - 20 reps

- Hold on to a dumbbell in front of you with both hands
- Squat down halfway so the dumbbell is between your legs – keep your back straight
- Power up from your buttocks and use momentum to swing the weight up to shoulder-height
- Swing back into a squat, keeping arms straight the whole time
- Keep momentum going for the entire set

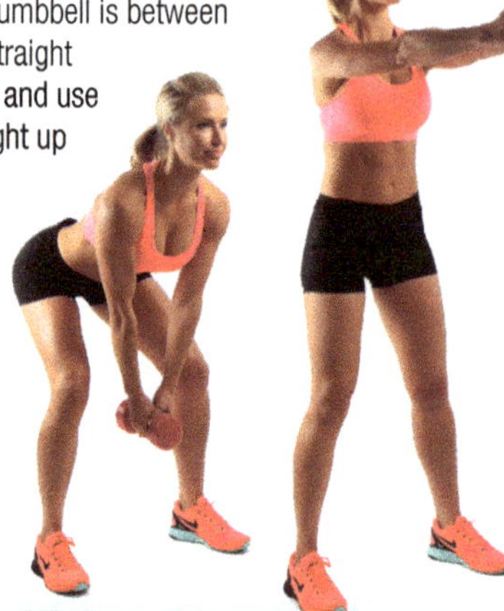

5 *Calf Raises* - 20 reps

- Holding dumbbells in each hand in a standing position, push up onto your toes by contracting your calves
- Hold for a second and return back down
- Do one foot at a time for an additional challenge
- For a deeper stretch, do on a step, making sure you hold on to something with one hand so you don't lose balance

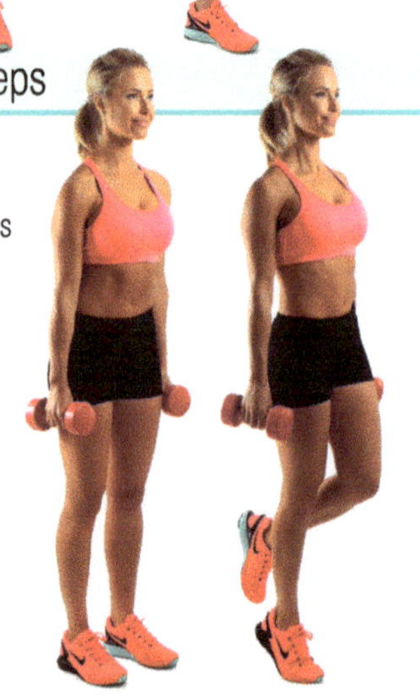

6 *Abs!* *Scissor Kicks* - 40 secs

- Lie on your back with your hands behind your head
- Lift both legs off the ground, then bring one leg up 90 degrees to your body
- Swap legs, keeping both legs straight throughout
- Keep your head off the ground by contracting your abs all the way

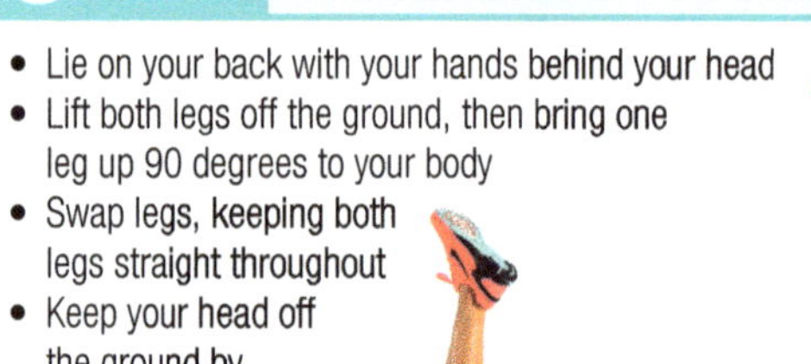

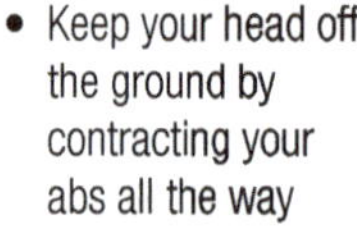

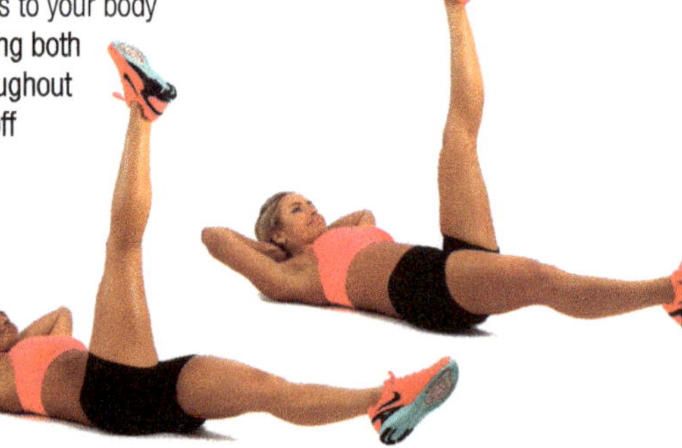

FAST WARMUP: 20 secs walk in place, 20 secs jog in place, 20 secs jumping jacks

LEAN HIIT BICEPS & TRICEPS

DAY 3

Equipment Workout bench or sofa + Dumbbells

Intervals Work - 40 seconds
Rest - 20 seconds

Rounds 24 rounds =
24 minutes in total

1 *Triceps Kickbacks* - 20 reps per side

- Bend over at the waist and rest your left hand and left knee on a bench
- With a dumbbell in your right hand, keep your elbow at your side, weight hanging down and extend your hand backwards
- Lower back to the starting position. Do 20 reps and change sides

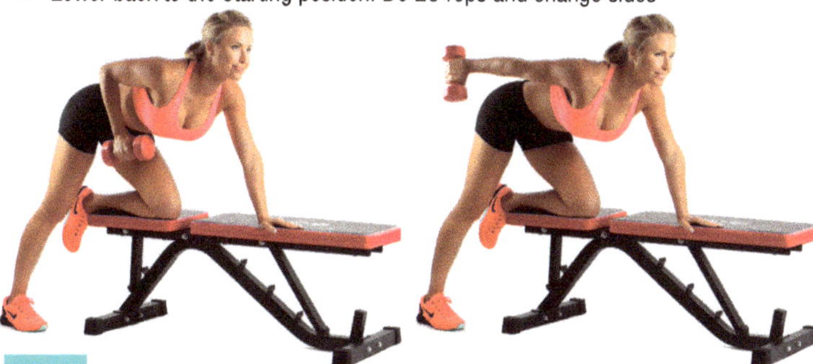

2 *Hammer Curls* - 20 reps

- Stand with dumbbells in each hand by your side, thumbs facing forward
- Lift up both dumbbells, keeping elbows by your sides
- Slowly lower the dumbbells in a 'hammer strike' motion, taking care not to swing the weights

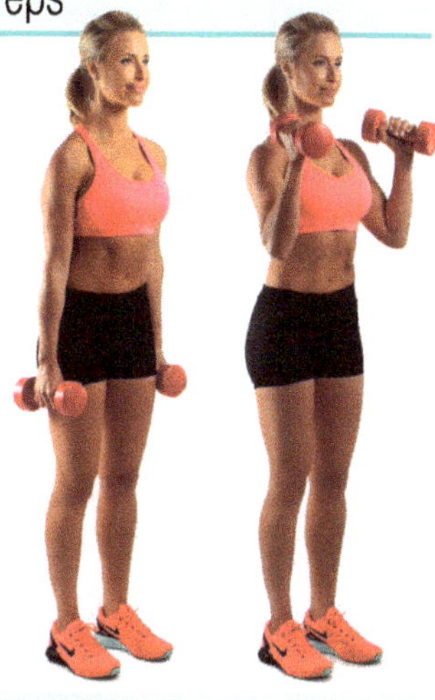

3 *Cardio Blast!* *Bench Step-ups* - 40 secs

- Stand in front of a bench (make sure it is stable and secure)
- Put your left foot on the bench and step up with your right leg
- Bring your right leg down again and swap legs

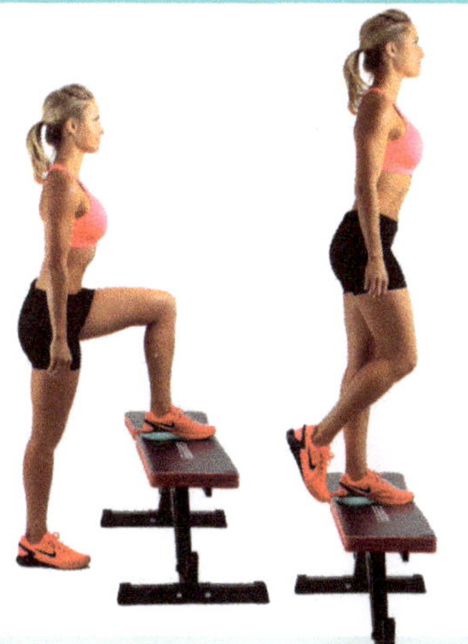

4 *Lying Triceps Extentions* - 20 reps

- Lying on your back on a bench, hold one dumbbell in both hands, stretched above your head
- Lower the weight by bending your elbows
- Bring the weight back to the starting position by contracting your triceps

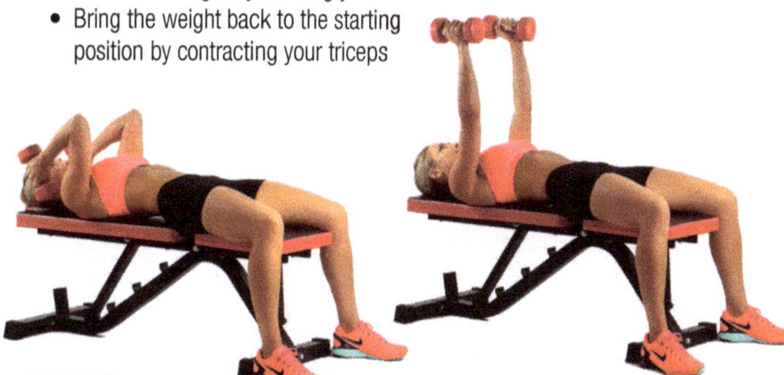

5 *Alternating Curls* - 20 reps

- In standing position, hold dumbbells in each hand hanging by your sides with thumbs facing outwards
- Lift up the weights by contracting your biceps, keeping your elbows by your side
- Slowly lower the dumbbells to the starting position, taking care not to swing the weights
- Make sure you do 20 reps with each arm

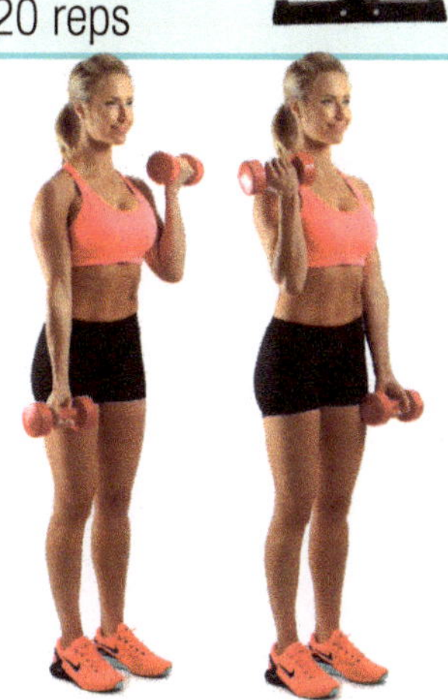

6 *Abs!* *Double Leg Lift* - 40 secs

- Lie on the floor with both hands by your side
- Keeping both legs straight, pivot at the waist and bring both legs up to 90 degrees, focusing on your abs contracting
- Slowly lower your legs back down and repeat

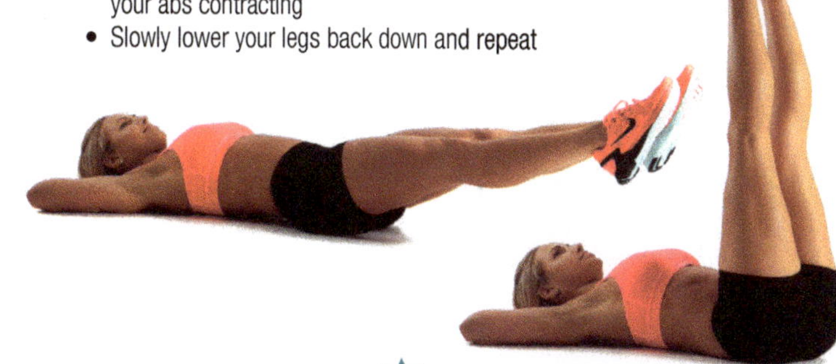

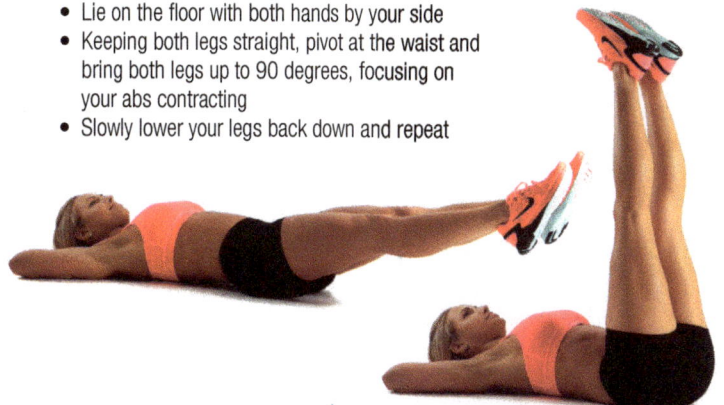

FAST WARMUP: 20 secs walk in place, 20 secs jog in place, 20 secs jumping jacks

4.4 Heavy HIIT

Looking for a body with more tone and definition? Then an athletic body is for you! This routine ups the weight to get a better response from your slow twitch muscle fibres to help you get a fantastically defined body, especially when you combine working out with our muscle-boosting food pyramids.

Developing an athletic body needs heavier weights as this gives your muscles the incentive to grow and has the added bonus of giving you an even faster metabolism as you add more muscle. All you need is 20 minutes a day, for four days a week!

Each workout is set up as a circuit - you do your reps over 40 seconds, rest for 20, then move on to the next exercise until you've reached the last exercise, and then start over again. This is going to keep you focused and your body challenged along the way.

Equipment needed

Even though we are going for heavier weights, you can still do all of these at home! You just need two pieces of equipment:

- **Adjustable dumbbells** – Get a pair of dumbbells that can go up to around 24kg (50lb) each. You probably won't need that much, but it's good to have it for when you get stronger! There are many types out there and they don't make a huge difference. Go out to a store, try some out and find a pair you like
- **Adjustable workout bench** – You can get one that folds up to easily store it, but make sure you get one since you'll need it!

Of course, you can also join a gym if you don't want to buy any equipment or if you like the energy of a gym. Personally I have everything at home so I don't have to drive all the way out to a gym to work out.

Heavy HIIT Workout Plan

Once again we have a workout that focuses on each body part, though this time we split it up between four groups:

1. **Chest and shoulders** – Pectorals and deltoids
2. **Back** – Upper back and latissimus dorsi
3. **Lower body** – Quadriceps, hamstrings, calves and gluteus maximus
4. **Arms** – Biceps and triceps

If you want to do more workouts in a week, add in Pure HIIT workouts for additional fat burning.

To give you a uniquely effective mix, each workout consists of three types of exercises:

1. **Primary muscle movers** – These directly target the muscle group you are going after for that day. For these exercises, use heavier weights so you can only do between 8 and 12 reps for a set. Lower the weight if you can't reach 8, or increase the weight if you can do more than 12
2. **Cardio blasts** – These get your heart racing for added fat burning effect. Do these for the full 40 seconds interval

3. **Abdominals** – Two of the workouts include abdominal exercises to get your core tight. Do these for the full 40 seconds interval

The workout formula goes like this:

1. *Do a quick 1 minute warmup – 20 seconds walking in place, 20 seconds jog in place, 20 seconds jumping jacks*
2. *Set your interval timer to 40 seconds 'Work' and 20 seconds 'Rest' for 20 rounds (total of 20 minutes)*
3. *Get started and do each of the exercises as indicated on the plans. Rest between each for 20 seconds and move on to the next exercise. Start back at the beginning when you've done all of them, for a total of 20 rounds.*
4. *Finish with a bit of stretching to cool down –* ***DONE!***

HEAVY HIIT CHEST & DELTOIDS

DAY 1

Sets and reps! Do 4 rounds of each exercise and use heavier weights so you can only do 8 to 12 reps of exercises 1, 3 & 4. Do exercises 2 & 5 for the full 40 seconds!

Equipment	Workout bench + Adjustable dumbbells
Intervals	Work - 40 seconds Rest - 20 seconds
Rounds	20 rounds = 20 minutes in total

1 *Chest Press*

- Lie on a bench and hold dumbbells in each hand just above your chest, keeping elbows pointed down
- Push the weights upwards, focusing on contracting your chest muscles
- Lower down to the starting position in a slow and controlled movement

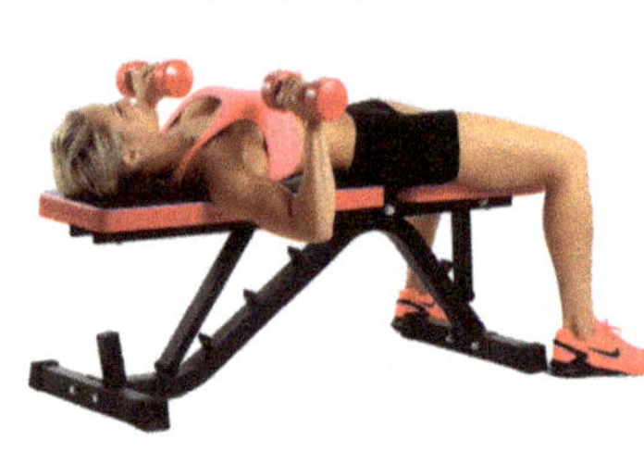

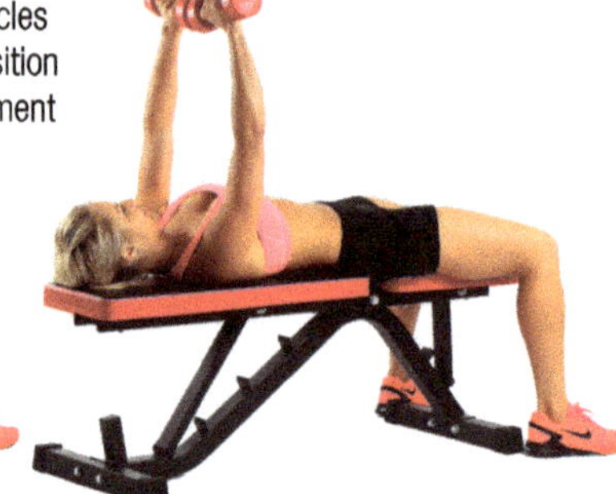

2 *Cardio Blast!* *Mountain Climbers*

- Start in a sprinting position
- Keeping hands on the ground, bring one knee into your chest while kicking the other leg back
- Keep going by swapping legs in a running motion

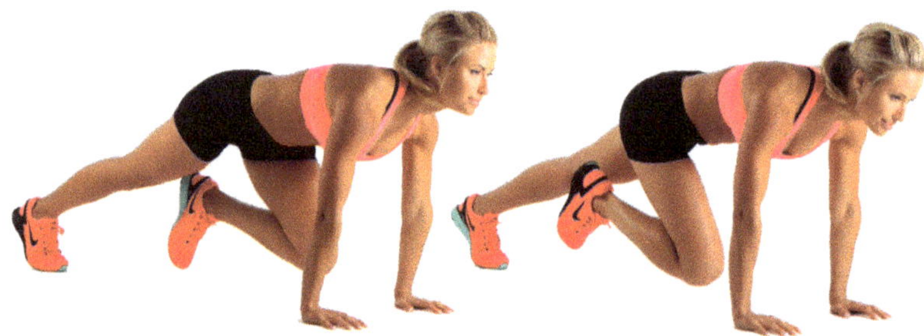

3 *Standing Shoulder Press*

- Start with dumbbells at shoulder height, thumbs facing backward
- Extend your arms upwards in a slow and controlled motion
- Bring back down to shoulder height

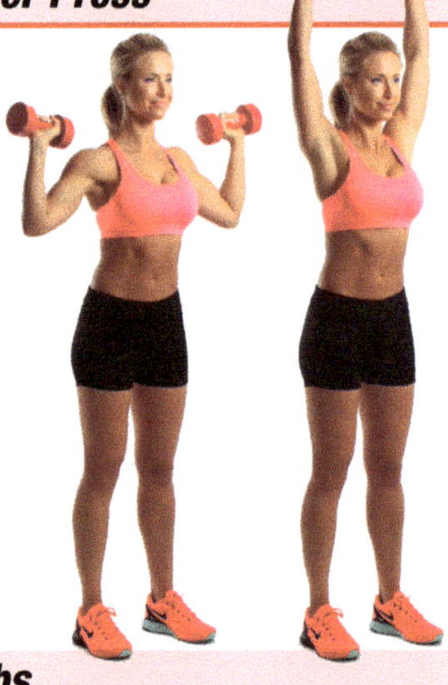

4 *Incline Press*

- Use an adjustable bench and set it on about a 30 degree incline
- Elbows pointing down, hold a dumbbell in each hand above your chest
- Push up and extend your arms upwards

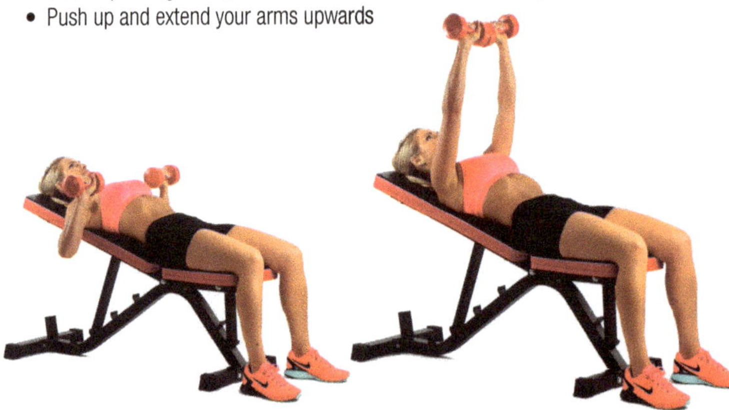

5 *Abs!* *Bicycle Abs*

- Lie on your back with your hands behind your head
- Lift up both legs and bring your left knee to your right elbow, contracting your abs
- Swap sides and keep going for the duration of the set

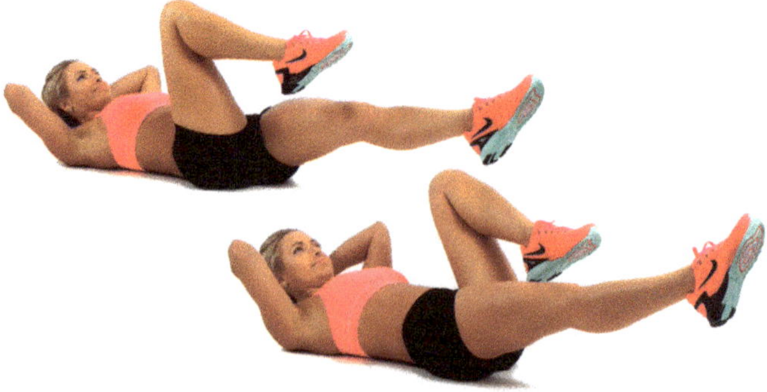

FAST WARMUP: 20 secs walk in place, 20 secs jog in place, 20 secs jumping jacks

HEAVY HIIT BACK WORKOUT

DAY 2

Sets and reps! Do 4 rounds of each exercise and use heavier weights so you can only do 8 to 12 reps of exercises 1, 3 & 4. Do exercises 2 & 5 for the full 40 seconds!

Equipment	Workout bench + Adjustable dumbbells
Intervals	Work - 40 seconds Rest - 20 seconds
Rounds	20 rounds = 20 minutes in total

1 Bent Over Rows

- Hold a dumbbell in each hand and bend over at the waist
- Pull up the dumbbells, keeping your elbows close to your sides
- Drop the weights back in front of you

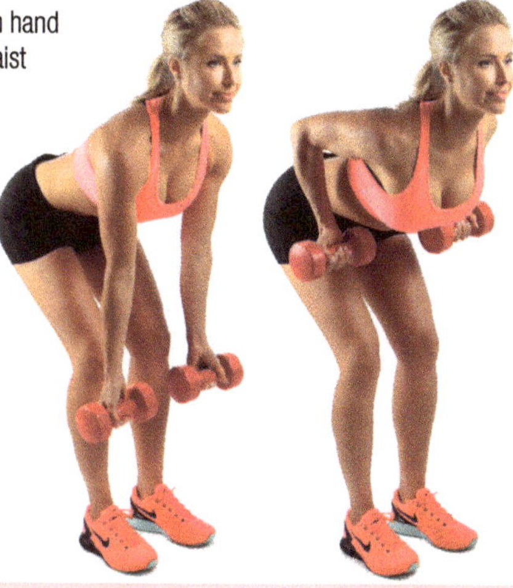

2 Cardio Blast! Side Lunge Jump

- Squat halfway down on one leg, hand touching the ground
- Point your other leg straight and off to the side
- Power up into a jump while bringing the outer leg in and pointing the inner leg out
- Jump while alternating between legs

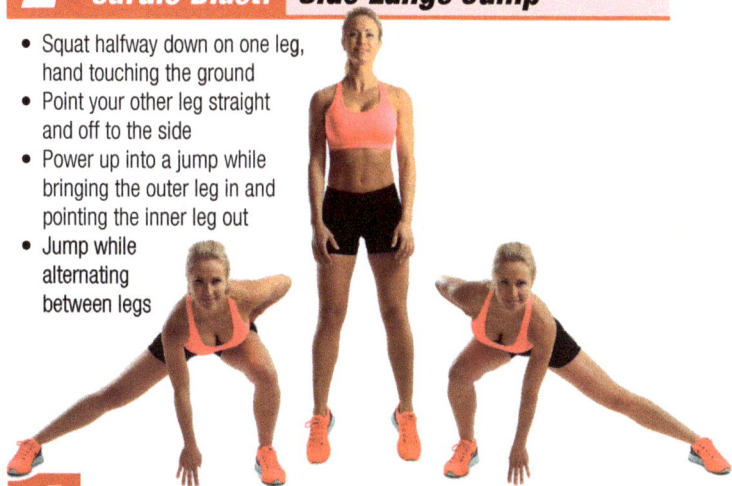

3 Dumbbell Reverse Flyes

- Hold dumbbells in each hand and bend over at the waist, keeping your back straight
- Keep your arms slightly bent and stiff, and swing them out to the sides, squeezing your shoulder blades
- Return to the starting position in a slow and controlled motion

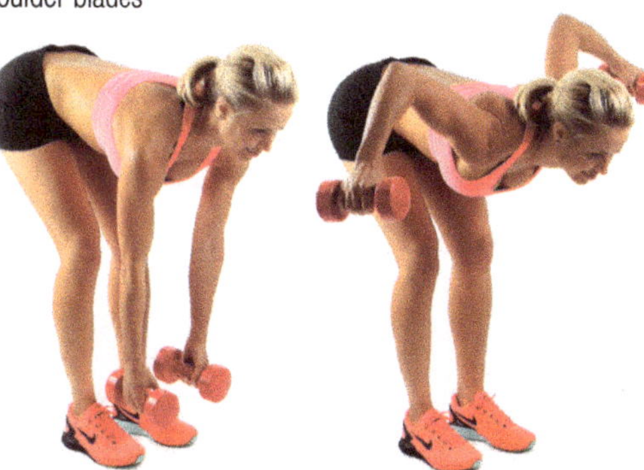

4 Pullovers

- Lying on your back on a bench, hold one dumbbell in both hands above your head
- Keeping your arms stiff and elbow slightly bent, lower the weight to behind your head by bending at your shoulders
- Raise the weight back to the starting position in a slow and controlled motion

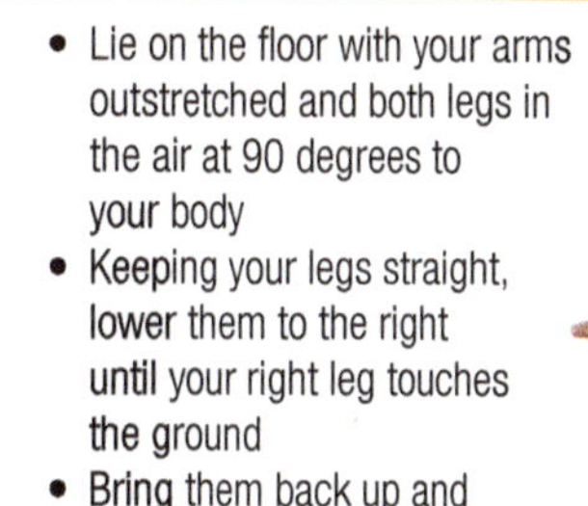

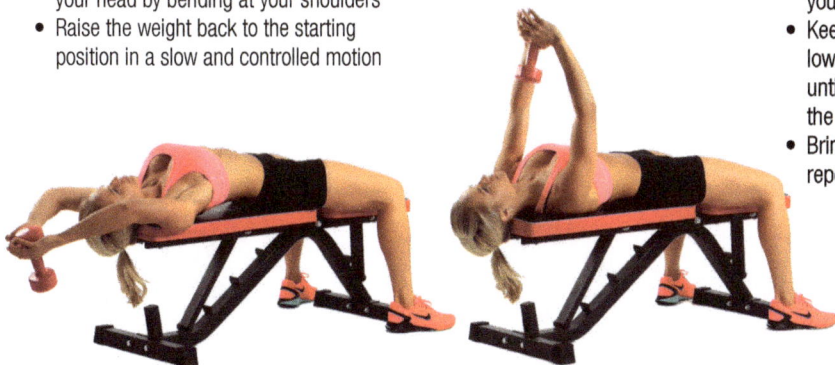

5 Abs! Windshield Wipers

- Lie on the floor with your arms outstretched and both legs in the air at 90 degrees to your body
- Keeping your legs straight, lower them to the right until your right leg touches the ground
- Bring them back up and repeat on the other side

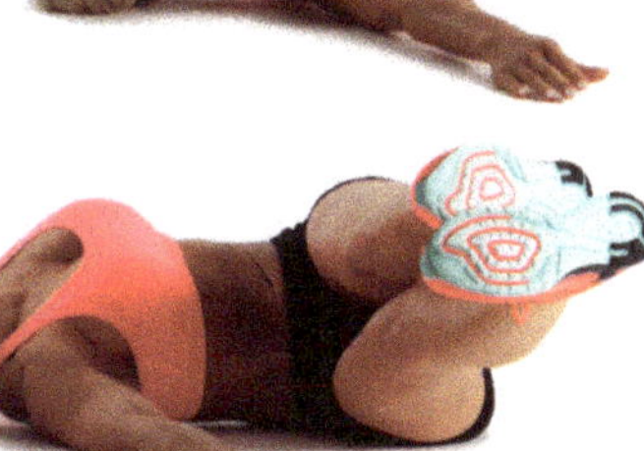

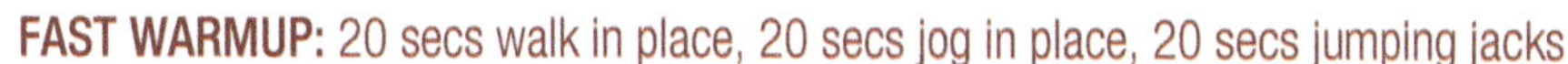

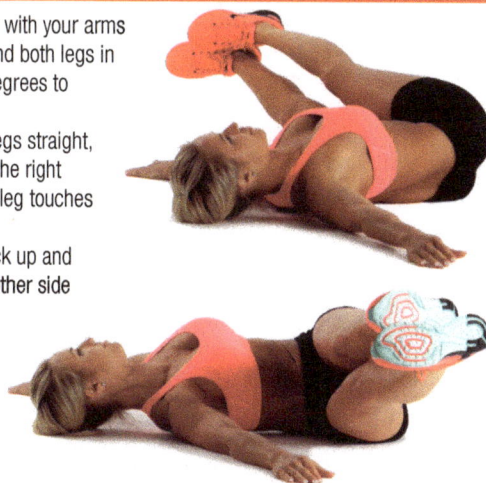

FAST WARMUP: 20 secs walk in place, 20 secs jog in place, 20 secs jumping jacks

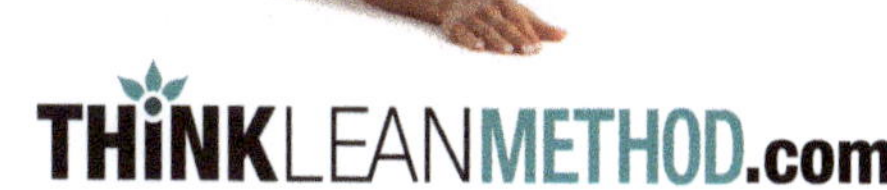

HEAVY HIIT LEGS & GLUTES

DAY 3

Sets and reps! Do 4 rounds of each exercise and use heavier weights so you can only do 8 to 12 reps of exercises 1, 2, 4 & 5. Do exercise 3 for the full 40 seconds!

Equipment	Workout bench + Adjustable dumbbells
Intervals	Work - 40 seconds Rest - 20 seconds
Rounds	20 rounds = 20 minutes in total

1 Goblet Squats

- Take one dumbbell in both hands and hold it close to your chest
- Squat down until your thighs are at least parallel to the floor, keeping your back straight
- Return to a standing position
- If you have access to a squat rack, do normal squats with a barbell on your shoulders

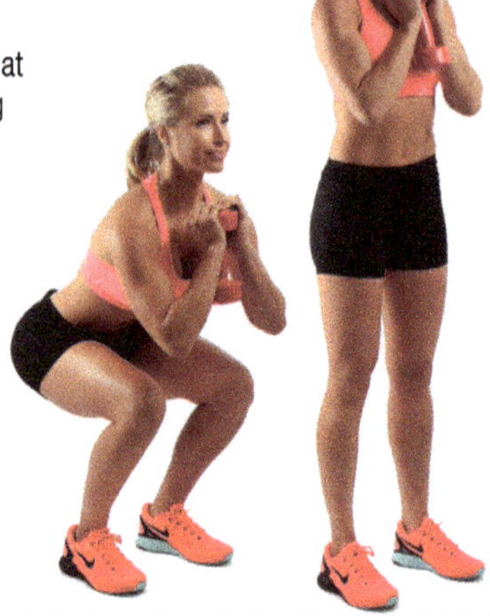

2 Calf Raises

- Holding dumbbells in each hand in a standing position, push up onto your toes by contracting your calves
- Hold for a second and return back down
- Do one foot at a time for an additional challenge
- For a deeper stretch, do on a step, making sure you hold on to something with one hand so you don't lose balance

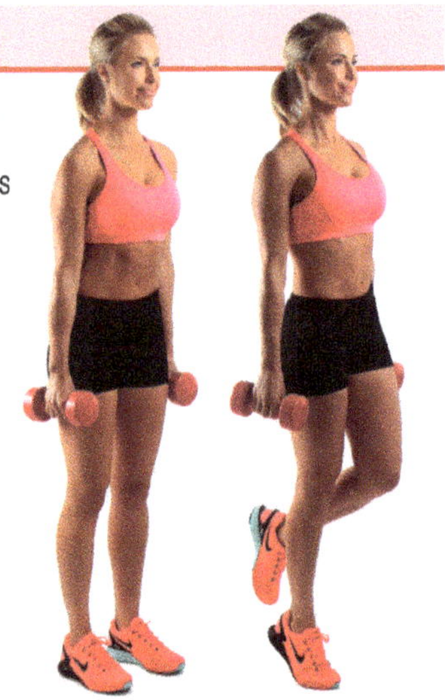

3 Cardio Blast! Bench Step-ups

- Stand in front of a bench (make sure it is stable and secure)
- Put your left foot on the bench and step up with your right leg
- Bring your right leg down again and swap legs

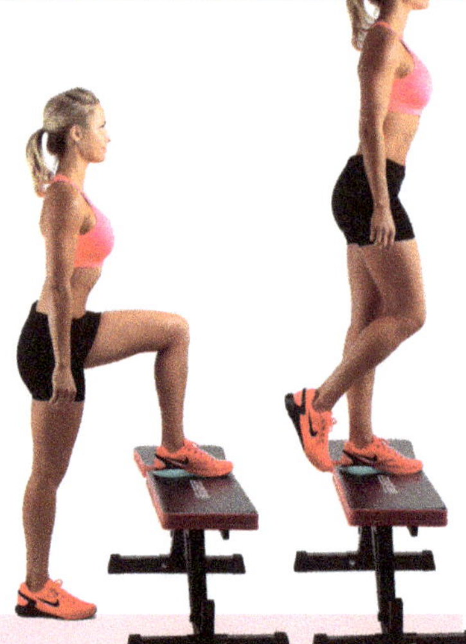

4 Stiff Leg Deadlifts

- Start in a standing position, holding dumbbells in each hand
- Keeping your back straight, bend over from the waist until you feel a stretch in the back of your legs
- Return to the starting position in a slow and controlled movement
- Do with a barbell if you have access to one

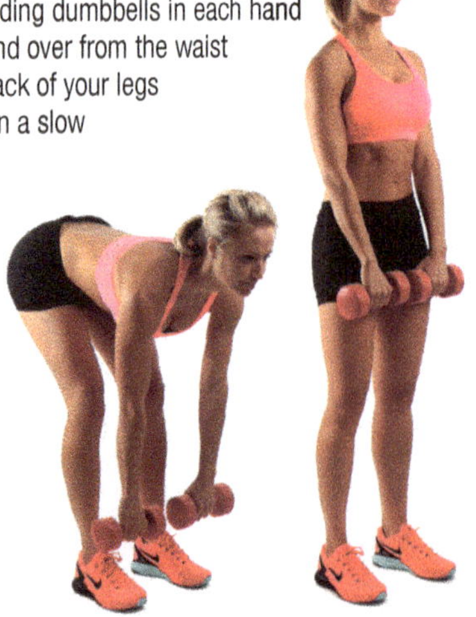

5 Hip Thrust

- Rest your shoulders on a bench, arms stretched out and hold on to stabilise yourself
- Keep one foot on the ground with knee bent at 90 degrees
- Hold the other leg in the air
- Drop down by bending at your waist and push back up until your body is parallel to the ground
- Do 20 reps and swap sides

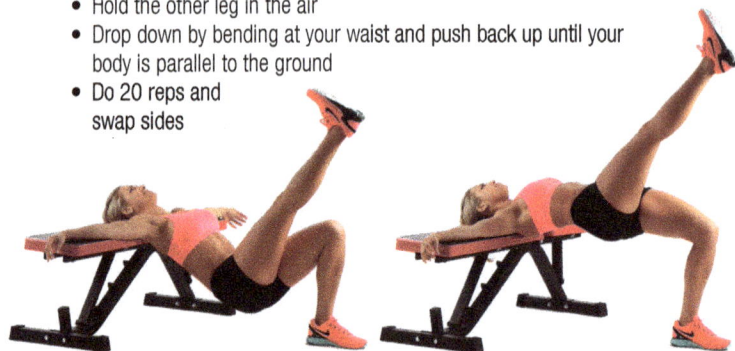

FAST WARMUP: 20 secs walk in place, 20 secs jog in place, 20 secs jumping jacks

HEAVY HIIT BICEPS & TRICEPS

DAY 4

Sets and reps! Do 4 rounds of each exercise and use heavier weights so you can only do 8 to 12 reps of exercises 1, 2, 4 & 5. Do exercise 3 for the full 40 seconds!

Equipment	Workout bench + Adjustable dumbbells
Intervals	Work - 40 seconds Rest - 20 seconds
Rounds	20 rounds = 20 minutes in total

1 *Triceps Kickbacks*

- Bend over at the waist and rest your left hand and left knee on a bench
- With a dumbbell in your right hand, keep your elbow at your side, weight hanging down
- Keeping your elbow still, extend your hand backwards until your triceps are fully extended
- Lower back to the starting position. Continue for one set then swap to the other hand

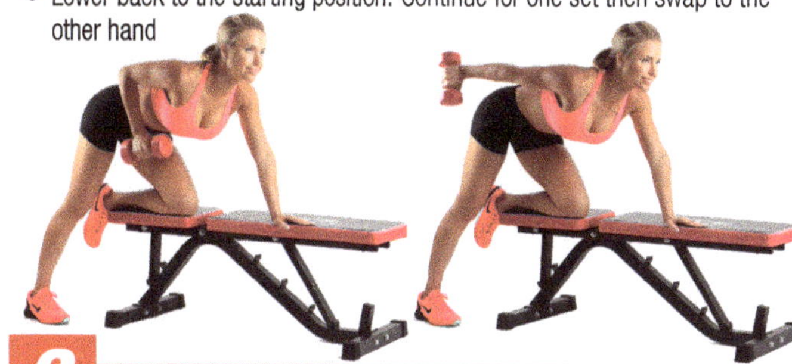

2 *Hammer Curls*

- Stand with dumbbells in each hand by your side, thumbs facing forward
- Lift up both dumbbells, keeping elbows by your sides
- Slowly lower the dumbbells in a 'hammer strike' motion, taking care not to swing the weights

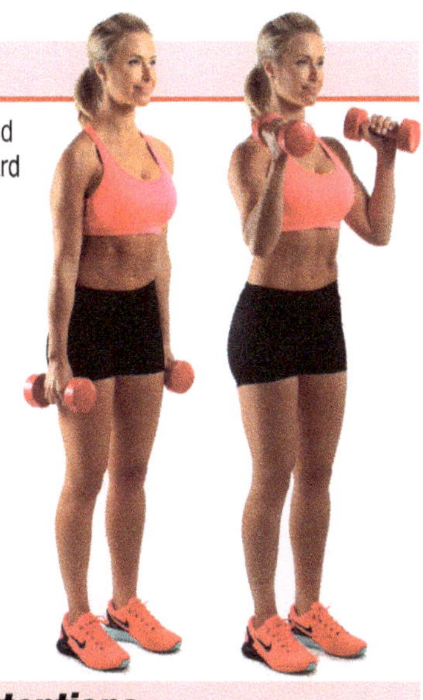

3 *Cardio Blast! High Knees Jog*

- Jog in place, each time driving up your knee as high as you can
- Keep up the pace for the full duration of the round
- Keep your core tight and chest up

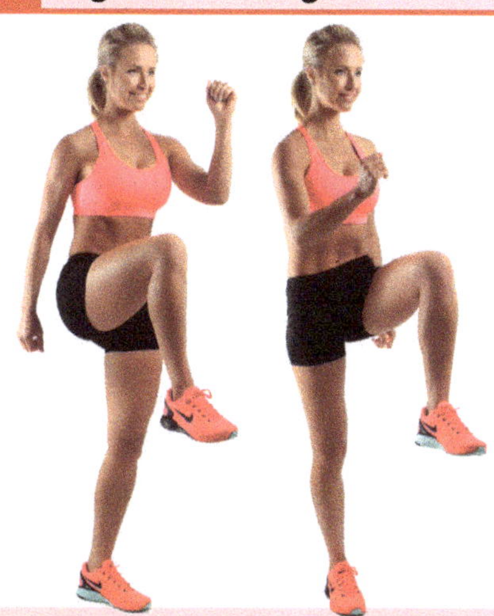

4 *Lying Triceps Extentions*

- Lying on your back on a bench, hold one dumbbell in both hands, stretched above your head
- Lower the weight by bending your elbows
- Bring the weight back to the starting position by contracting your triceps

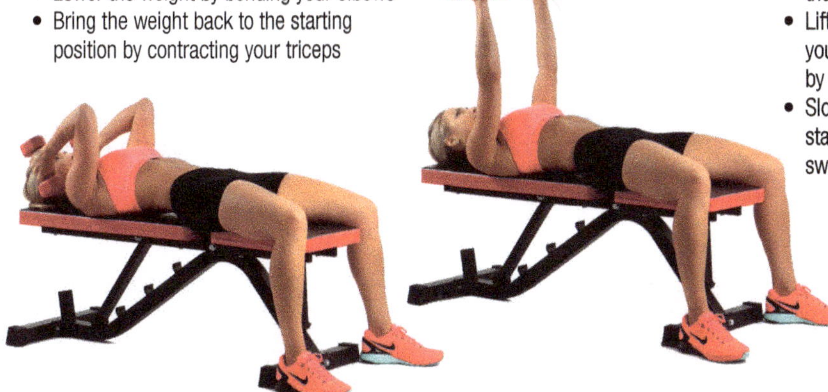

5 *Alternating Curls*

- In standing position, hold dumbbells in each hand hanging by your sides with thumbs facing outwards
- Lift up the weights by contracting your biceps, keeping your elbows by your side
- Slowly lower the dumbbells to the starting position, taking care not to swing the weights

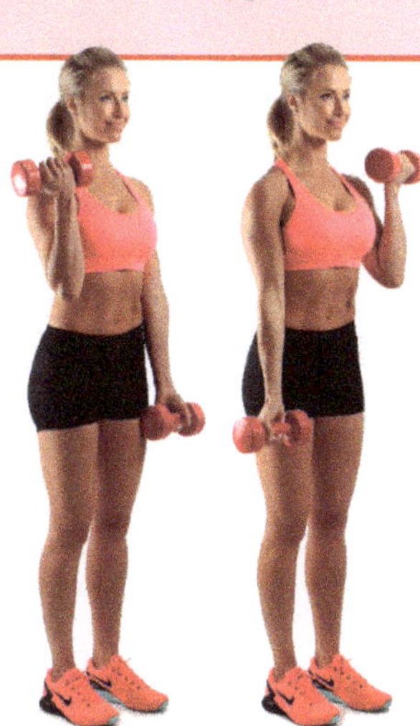

FAST WARMUP: 20 secs walk in place, 20 secs jog in place, 20 secs jumping jacks

THiNKLEANMETHOD

TRACKING SHEET

Tick off your progress towards your goals every day, then start a new sheet every three months when it's filled. You can tick each box where you stuck to the plan. If you cheated (anything off plan), then mark that box with an 'X' and make a note of what you ate. This will help you diagnose what's going wrong if you don't progress to your goal. Remember to take photos as well, weigh yourself and measure every two weeks.

Five basic nutrition rules

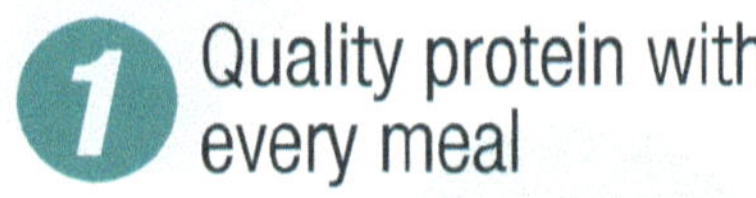

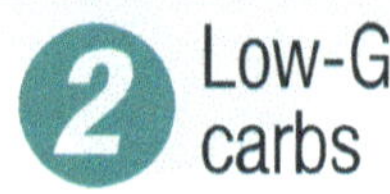

3 Whole foods

4 Mix it up

5 Slow down

Prioritised goals

Specific, measurable, attainable, **relevant** & timeframe

Write the nutrition plan and workout plan you will do over the next three months

1. ______________________________
2. ______________________________
3. ______________________________
4. ______________________________
5. ______________________________

Personal vision

Broad, positive characteristics to become

Write here the type of body you want to achieve or maintain

1. ______________________________
2. ______________________________
3. ______________________________
4. ______________________________
5. ______________________________

	S	M	T	W	T	F	S	S	M	T	W	T	F	S	**Weight / Waist**			S	M	T	W	T	F	S	S	M	T	W	T	F	S	**Weight / Waist**	
Month 1																	➤																
Month 2																	➤																
Month 3																	➤																

☑ Tick each day that you stayed consistent with your eating plan.

THiNK LEAN METHOD

Starting weight and waist measurement		
Start date of this sheet		

Next Steps!

- **Take new pictures**
- **Start the next sheet**

THiNK LEAN METHOD

CORE ACM Food Pyramid

Fruit

Stick to one a day or less

- Apples
- Apricots
- Avocados
- Bananas
- Blackberries
- Blueberries
- Cherries
- Cranberries
- Date
- Dragonfruit
- Grapefruit
- Grapes
- Guavas
- Kiwis
- Kumquat
- Lemons
- Limes
- Luquat
- Lychees
- Mandarins
- Mangoes
- Mangosteen
- Melons
- Mulberry
- Nectarines
- Olives
- Oranges
- Papayas
- Passionfruit
- Peaches
- Pears
- Pineapples
- Plums
- Pomegranates
- Raspberries
- Rhubarb
- Star fruit
- Strawberries
- Tangerines
- Watermelon

Vegetables

The more you eat, the better!

- Alfalfa seeds
- Amaranth
- Artichoke
- Asparagus
- Bamboo shoots
- Bell peppers
- Bok choi
- Broccoli
- Brussels sprouts
- Butternut squash
- Cabbage
- Carrots
- Cauliflower
- Celery
- Chicory
- Chilli
- Chinese broccoli
- Chinese cabbage
- Collard greens
- Cucumber
- Eggplant
- Fennel
- Gem Squash
- Green beans
- Green onions
- Jalapeno peppers
- Kale
- Leeks
- Lettuce (various)
- Mushrooms (various)
- Okra
- Onions
- Parsley
- Radishes
- Rhubarb
- Sauerkraut
- Scallions
- Seaweed
- Spaghetti squash
- Spinach
- Swiss chard
- Tomatoes
- Turnips
- Watercress
- Zucchini
- Daikon
- Snap peas

LG

Nuts & Oils

Snacks & small amounts

Nuts

- Almonds
- Brazil nuts
- Cashews
- Chestnuts
- Coconut
- Hazelnuts
- Macadamia
- Peacan
- Peanuts
- Pine nuts
- Pistachio
- Wallnuts

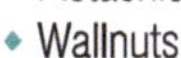

Oils & Fats

- Butter
- Ghee
- Coconut oil
- Tallow
- Lard
- Avocado oil
- Almond oil

Dairy

One portion a day

- Milk (full cream)
- Cheddar
- Gouda
- Swiss cheese
- Cottage cheese
- Parmesan
- Edam
- Mozzarella
- Fat-free cheese
- Whey
- Yoghurt (sugar free)

Fruit

Nuts & Oils

Dairy
No added sugar

Vegetables
Low-GI, non-starchy

Meat, Poultry, Fish, Eggs
Lean meats, no visible dietary fat

Core ACM

Meat, Poultry, Fish, Eggs

Eat most of - lean protein with every meal

Poultry

- Chicken
- Duck
- Goose
- Ostrich
- Quail
- Turkey
- All eggs

Lean cuts like:

- Breast
- Tenderloin

Meat

- Beef
- Kangaroo
- Lamb
- Pork
- Rabbit
- Veal
- Wild meat

Lean cuts like:

- 95% mince
- Sirloin
- Tenderloin
- Lean bacon

Fish

- Anchovy
- Herring
- John Dory
- Mackerel
- Mullet
- Octopus
- Salmon
- Sardines
- Snapper
- Squid
- Trout
- Tuna
- Whiting

Shellfish

- Clams
- Crab
- Lobster
- Mussels
- Oysters
- Prawns
- Scallops

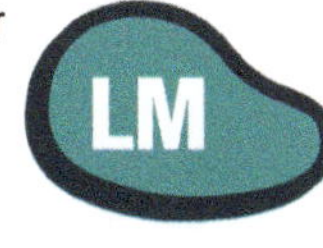

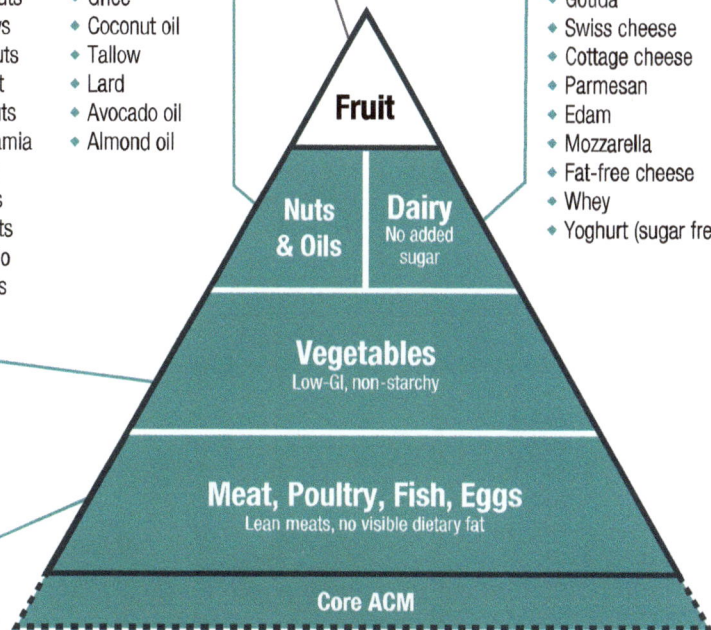

THiNK LEAN METHOD

Herbs & Spices

Use as much seasoning as you like!

- Angelica
- Anise
- Basil
- Bay leaf
- Caraway
- Cardamom
- Carob
- Cayenne pepper
- Celery seed
- Chervil
- Chili pepper
- Chives
- Cilantro
- Cinnamon
- Clove
- Coriander
- Cumin
- Curry
- Dill
- Fennel
- Fenugreek
- Galangal
- Garlic
- Ginger
- Horseradish
- Jasmine flowers
- Juniper berry
- Kaffir lime leaves
- Lavender
- Lemongrass
- Licorice
- Mace
- Marjoram
- Mint
- Mustard
- Nutmeg
- Oregano
- Paprika
- Parseley
- Pepper
- Peppermint
- Rosemary
- Saffron
- Sage
- Salt
- Sesame
- Star anise
- Tarragon
- Thyme
- Turmeric
- Vanilla
- Wasabi
- Wattleseed
- Za'atar

* This is not an exhaustive list! If you find foods that fit with the rules that are not on here, add them in!

THINK LEAN METHOD

COMPLETE ACM Food Pyramid

Fruit

Stick to one a day or less

- Apples
- Apricots
- Avocados
- Bananas
- Blackberries
- Blueberries
- Cherries
- Cranberries
- Date
- Dragonfruit
- Grapefruit
- Grapes
- Guavas
- Kiwis
- Kumquat
- Lemons
- Limes
- Luquat
- Lychees
- Mandarins
- Mangoes
- Mangosteen
- Melons
- Mulberry
- Nectarines
- Olives
- Oranges
- Papayas
- Passionfruit
- Peaches
- Pears
- Pineapples
- Plums
- Pomegranates
- Raspberries
- Rhubarb
- Star fruit
- Strawberries
- Tangerines
- Watermelon

Vegetables

Low-GI - The more the better!

- Alfalfa seeds
- Amaranth
- Artichoke
- Asparagus
- Bamboo shoots
- Bell peppers
- Bok choi
- Broccoli
- Brussels sprouts
- Butternut squash
- Cabbage
- Carrots
- Cauliflower
- Celery
- Chicory
- Chilli
- Chinese broccoli
- Chinese cabbage
- Collard greens
- Cucumber
- Eggplant
- Fennel
- Gem Squash
- Green beans
- Green onions
- Jalapeno peppers
- Kale
- Leeks
- Lettuce (various)
- Mushrooms (various)
- Okra
- Onions
- Parsley
- Radishes
- Rhubarb
- Sauerkraut
- Scallions
- Seaweed
- Spaghetti squash
- Spinach
- Swiss chard
- Tomatoes
- Turnips
- Watercress
- Zucchini
- Daikon
- Snap peas

LG

Nuts & Oils

Snacks & small amounts

Nuts

- Almonds
- Cashews
- Coconut
- Hazelnuts
- Macadamia
- Peacan
- Peanuts
- Pistachio
- Wallnuts

Oils & Fats

- Butter
- Ghee
- Coconut oil
- Avocado oil
- Almond oil

Dairy

One portion a day

- Milk (full cream)
- Cheddar
- Gouda
- Swiss cheese
- Cottage cheese
- Parmesan
- Edam
- Mozzarella
- Fat-free cheese
- Whey
- Yoghurt (sugar free)

Legumes

Snacks & small amounts

- Black beans
- Broad beans
- Butter beans
- Chickpeas
- Edamame
- Kidney beans
- Lentils
- Peas
- Soy beans
- Split peas

Veggies

Starchy for fuel

- Beets
- Plantains
- Pumpkin
- Sweet corn
- Sweet potato
- Waterchestnuts
- Yam

SV

Fruit

Nuts & Oils

Dairy
No added sugar

Leg-umes

Vegetables
Low-GI, non-starchy

Veggies
Starchy

Meat, Poultry, Fish, Eggs
Lean meats, no visible dietary fat

Fatty Meats
Visible dietary fat

Complete ACM - Includes all Core ACM foods (regular exercise)

LM

Meat, Poultry, Fish, Eggs

Eat most of - lean protein with every meal

Poultry

- Chicken
- Duck
- Goose
- Ostrich
- Quail
- Turkey
- All eggs

Lean cuts like:

- Breast
- Tenderloin

Meat

- Beef
- Kangaroo
- Lamb
- Pork
- Rabbit
- Veal
- Wild meat

Lean cuts like:

- 95% ground beef
- Sirloin
- Tenderloin
- Lean bacon

Fish

- Anchovy
- Herring
- John Dory
- Mackerel
- Mullet
- Octopus
- Salmon
- Sardines
- Snapper
- Squid
- Trout
- Tuna
- Whiting

Shellfish

- Clams
- Crab
- Lobster
- Mussels
- Oysters
- Prawns
- Scallops

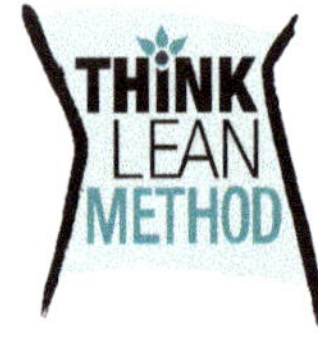

Herbs & Spices

Use as much seasoning as you like!

- Angelica
- Anise
- Basil
- Bay leaf
- Caraway
- Cardamom
- Carob
- Cayenne pepper
- Celery seed
- Chervil
- Chili pepper
- Chives
- Cilantro
- Cinnamon
- Clove
- Coriander
- Cumin
- Curry
- Dill
- Fennel
- Fenugreek
- Galangal
- Garlic
- Ginger
- Horseradish
- Jasmine flowers
- Juniper berry
- Kaffir lime leaves
- Lavender
- Lemongrass
- Licorice
- Mace
- Marjoram
- Mint
- Mustard
- Nutmeg
- Oregano
- Paprika
- Parseley
- Pepper
- Peppermint
- Rosemary
- Saffron
- Sage
- Salt
- Sesame
- Star anise
- Tarragon
- Thyme
- Turmeric
- Vanilla
- Wasabi
- Wattleseed
- Za'atar

Meats

Fatty cuts for fuel

Poultry

- Drumstick
- Leg quarter
- Poultry with skin on
- Thigh

Meat

- New York Strip
- Porterhouse steak
- Ribeye steak
- Ribs
- T-bone steak
- Wagyu
- Chops
- Bacon

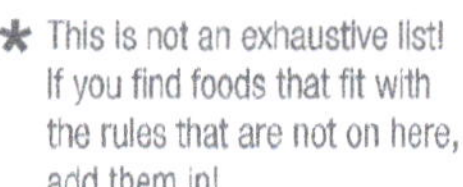

* This is not an exhaustive list! If you find foods that fit with the rules that are not on here, add them in!

THiNK LEAN METHOD

THINK FREE Food Pyramid

Fruit

Stick to one a day or less

- Apples
- Apricots
- Avocados
- Bananas
- Blackberries
- Blueberries
- Cherries
- Cranberries
- Date
- Dragonfruit
- Grapefruit
- Grapes
- Guavas
- Kiwis
- Kumquat
- Lemons
- Limes
- Luquat
- Lychees
- Mandarins
- Mangoes
- Mangosteen
- Melons
- Mulberry
- Nectarines
- Olives
- Oranges
- Papayas
- Passionfruit
- Peaches
- Pears
- Pineapples
- Plums
- Pomegranates
- Raspberries
- Rhubarb
- Star fruit
- Strawberries
- Tangerines
- Watermelon

Meat, Poultry, Fish, Eggs

Eat lean sources of meal with most meals to help optimise insulin response

Poultry

- Chicken
- Duck
- Goose
- Ostrich
- Quail
- Turkey
- All eggs

Lean cuts like:

- Breast
- Tenderloin

Meat

- Beef
- Kangaroo
- Lamb
- Pork
- Rabbit
- Veal
- Wild meat

Lean cuts like:

- 95% ground beef
- Sirloin
- Tenderloin

Fish

- Anchovy
- Herring
- John Dory
- Mackerel
- Mullet
- Octopus
- Salmon
- Sardines
- Snapper
- Squid
- Trout
- Tuna
- Whiting

Shellfish

- Clams
- Crab
- Lobster
- Mussels
- Oysters
- Prawns
- Scallops

LM

Nuts & Oils

Snacks & small amounts

Nuts

- Almonds
- Cashews
- Coconut
- Hazelnuts
- Macadamia
- Peacan
- Peanuts
- Pistachio
- Wallnuts

Oils & Fats

- Butter
- Ghee
- Coconut oil
- Avocado oil
- Almond oil

Dairy

One portion a day

- Milk (full cream)
- Cheddar
- Gouda
- Swiss cheese
- Cottage cheese
- Parmesan
- Edam
- Mozzarella
- Fat-free cheese
- Whey
- Yoghurt (sugar free)

Legumes

One portion a day

- Black beans
- Broad beans
- Butter beans
- Chickpeas
- Edamame
- Kidney beans
- Lentils
- Peas
- Soy beans
- Split peas

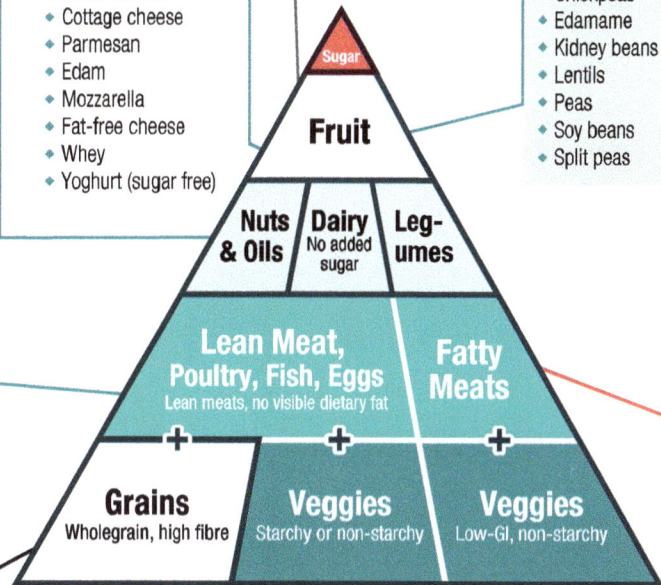

Sugar

Fruit

Nuts & Oils | Dairy No added sugar | Leg-umes

Lean Meat, Poultry, Fish, Eggs
Lean meats, no visible dietary fat

Fatty Meats

Grains
Wholegrain, high fibre

Veggies
Starchy or non-starchy

Veggies
Low-GI, non-starchy

Whole Grains

Control portion sizes

- Rolled oats
- Brown rice
- Barley
- Quinoa
- Buckwheat
- Semolina

WG

Stick to whole foods, but these can work if you control portions sizes:

- Wholewheat pasta
- Wholewheat bread
- Sourdough
- Rye bread

Veggies

Starchy for fuel

- Beets
- Plantains
- Pumpkin
- Sweet corn
- Sweet potato
- Waterchestnuts
- Yam

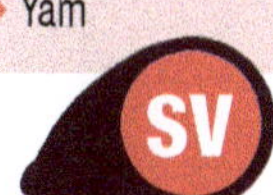

Low-GI Veggies

The more the better!

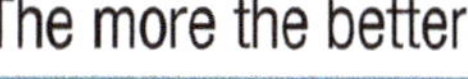

LG

- Alfalfa seeds
- Amaranth
- Artichoke
- Asparagus
- Bamboo shoots
- Bell peppers
- Bok choi
- Broccoli
- Brussels sprouts
- Butternut squash
- Cabbage
- Carrots
- Cauliflower
- Celery
- Chicory
- Chilli
- Chinese broccoli
- Chinese cabbage
- Collard greens
- Cucumber
- Eggplant
- Fennel
- Gem Squash
- Green beans
- Green onions
- Jalapeno peppers
- Kale
- Leeks
- Lettuce (various)
- Mushrooms
- Okra
- Onions
- Parsley
- Radishes
- Rhubarb
- Sauerkraut
- Scallions
- Seaweed
- Spaghetti squash
- Spinach
- Swiss chard
- Tomatoes
- Turnips
- Watercress
- Zucchini
- Daikon
- Snap peas

Meats

Fatty cuts for fuel

Poultry

- Drumstick
- Leg quarter
- Poultry with skin on
- Thigh

Meat

- New York Strip
- Porterhouse steak
- Ribeye steak
- Ribs
- T-bone steak
- Wagyu
- Chops
- Bacon

* This is not an exhaustive list! If you find foods that fit with the rules that are not on here, add them in!

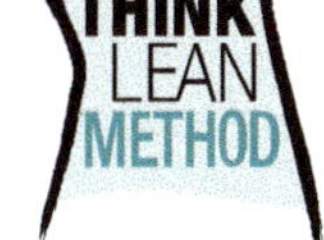

Herbs & Spices

Use as much seasoning as you like!

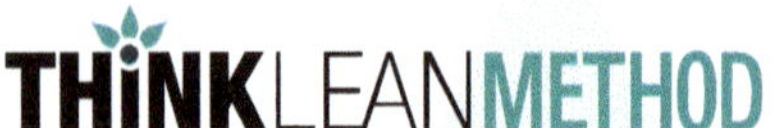

THINK BIG
Food Pyramid

Fruit
Stick to one a day or less

- Apples
- Apricots
- Avocados
- Bananas
- Blackberries
- Blueberries
- Cherries
- Cranberries
- Date
- Dragonfruit
- Grapefruit
- Grapes
- Guavas
- Kiwis
- Kumquat
- Lemons
- Limes
- Luquat
- Lychees
- Mandarins
- Mangoes
- Mangosteen
- Melons
- Mulberry
- Nectarines
- Olives
- Oranges
- Papayas
- Passionfruit
- Peaches
- Pears
- Pineapples
- Plums
- Pomegranates
- Raspberries
- Rhubarb
- Star fruit
- Strawberries
- Tangerines
- Watermelon

Vegetables
Low-GI - The more the better!

- Alfalfa seeds
- Amaranth
- Artichoke
- Asparagus
- Bamboo shoots
- Bell peppers
- Bok choi
- Broccoli
- Brussels sprouts
- Butternut squash
- Cabbage
- Carrots
- Cauliflower
- Celery
- Chicory
- Chilli
- Chinese broccoli
- Chinese cabbage
- Collard greens
- Cucumber
- Eggplant
- Fennel
- Gem Squash
- Green beans
- Green onions
- Jalapeno peppers
- Kale
- Leeks
- Lettuce (various)
- Mushrooms (various)
- Okra
- Onions
- Parsley
- Radishes
- Rhubarb
- Sauerkraut
- Scallions
- Seaweed
- Spaghetti squash
- Spinach
- Swiss chard
- Tomatoes
- Turnips
- Watercress
- Zucchini
- Daikon
- Snap peas

LG

Nuts & Oils
Snacks & small amounts

Nuts
- Almonds
- Cashews
- Coconut
- Hazelnuts
- Macadamia
- Peacan
- Peanuts
- Pistachio
- Wallnuts

Oils & Fats
- Butter
- Ghee
- Coconut oil
- Avocado oil
- Almond oil

Dairy
Small amounts

- Milk (full cream)
- Cheddar
- Gouda
- Swiss cheese
- Cottage cheese
- Parmesan
- Edam
- Mozzarella
- Fat-free cheese
- Whey
- Yoghurt (sugar free)

Legumes
One portion a day

- Black beans
- Broad beans
- Butter beans
- Chickpeas
- Edamame
- Kidney beans
- Lentils
- Peas
- Soy beans
- Split peas

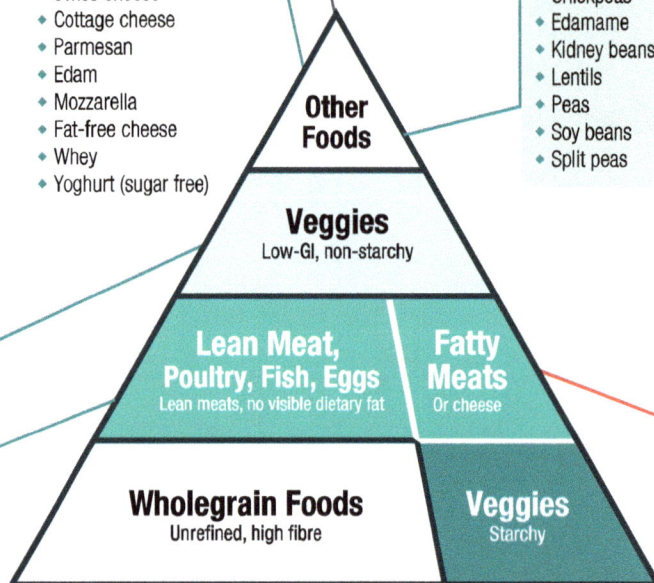

Other Foods

Veggies
Low-GI, non-starchy

Lean Meat, Poultry, Fish, Eggs
Lean meats, no visible dietary fat

Fatty Meats
Or cheese

Wholegrain Foods
Unrefined, high fibre

Veggies
Starchy

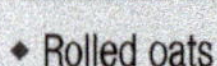

Meat, Poultry, Fish, Eggs
Eat most of - lean protein with every meal

Poultry
- Chicken
- Duck
- Goose
- Ostrich
- Quail
- Turkey
- All eggs

Lean cuts like:
- Breast
- Tenderloin

Meat
- Beef
- Kangaroo
- Lamb
- Pork
- Rabbit
- Veal
- Wild meat

Lean cuts like:
- 95% ground beef
- Sirloin
- Tenderloin
- Lean bacon

Fish
- Anchovy
- Herring
- John Dory
- Mackerel
- Mullet
- Octopus
- Salmon
- Sardines
- Snapper
- Squid
- Trout
- Tuna
- Whiting

Shellfish
- Clams
- Crab
- Lobster
- Mussels
- Oysters
- Prawns
- Scallops

THINK LEAN METHOD

Whole Grains
Have plenty

- Rolled oats
- Brown rice
- Barley
- Quinoa
- Buckwheat
- Semolina

Stick to whole foods, but these can work if you control portions sizes:

- Wholewheat pasta
- Wholewheat bread
- Sourdough
- Rye bread

WG

Veggies
Starchy for fuel

- Beets
- Plantains
- Pumpkin
- Sweet corn
- Sweet potato
- Waterchestnuts
- Yam

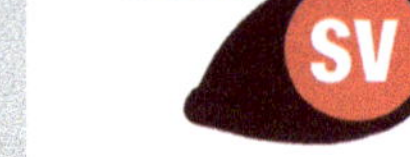

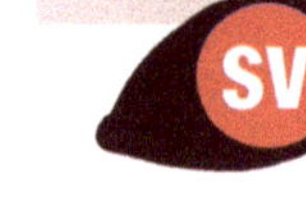

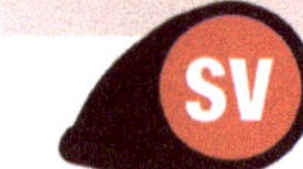

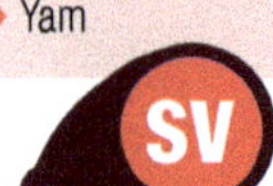

Meats
Fatty cuts for fuel

Poultry
- Drumstick
- Leg quarter
- Poultry with skin on
- Thigh

Meat
- New York Strip
- Porterhouse steak
- Ribeye steak
- Ribs
- T-bone steak
- Wagyu
- Chops
- Bacon

FM

Herbs & Spices
Use as much seasoning as you like!

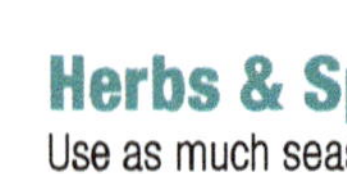

★ This is not an exhaustive list! If you find foods that fit with the rules that are not on here, add them in!

Portion Guidelines

Each of the sections on this page list how much is usually contained in one serving of that food type. Refer to the individual nutrition plans for how many servings to eat of each food type per day.

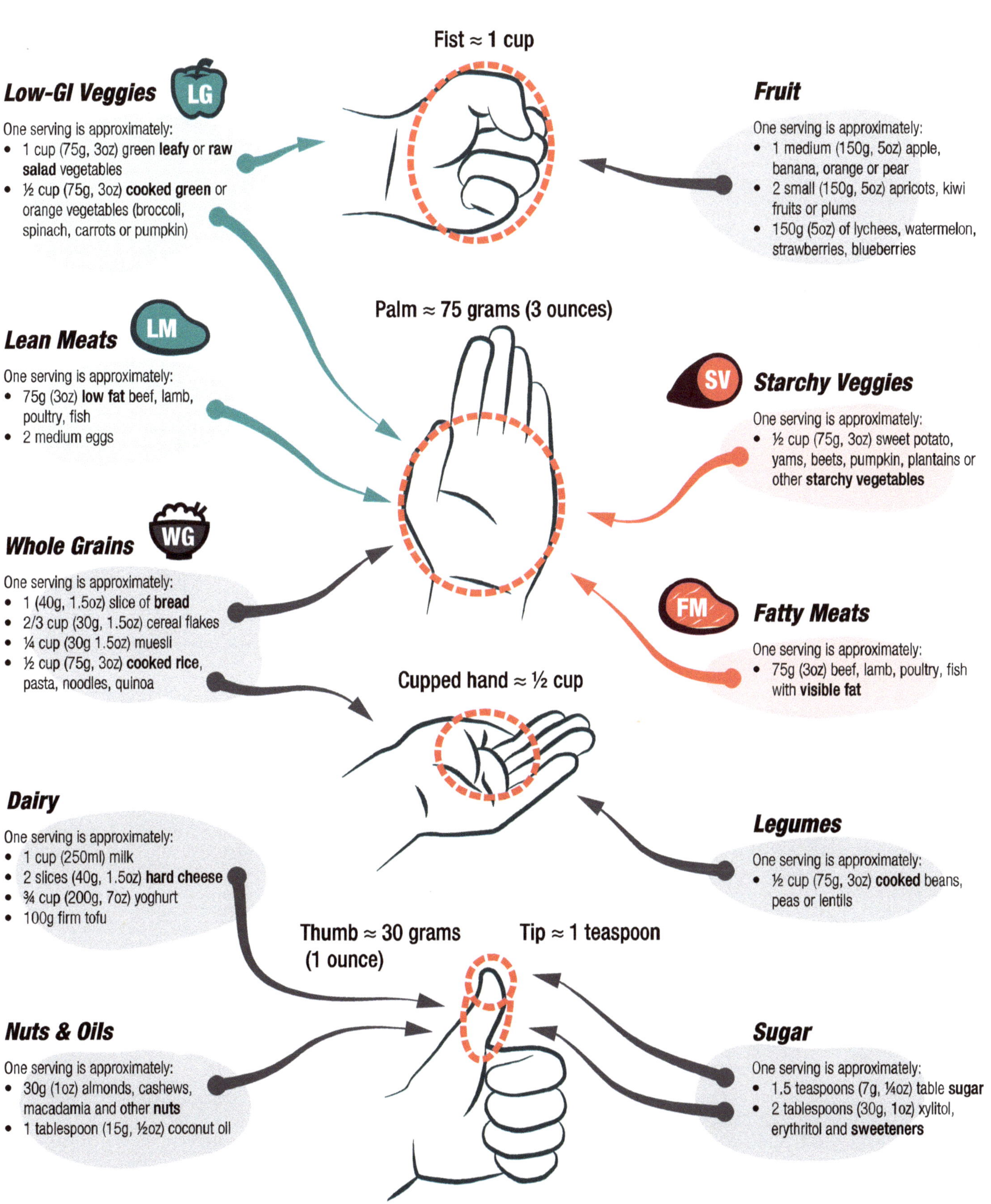

Fist ≈ 1 cup
Low-GI Veggies
LG
One serving is approximately:
• 1 cup (75g, 3oz) green **leafy** or **raw salad** vegetables
• ½ cup (75g, 3oz) **cooked green** or orange vegetables (broccoli, spinach, carrots or pumpkin)
Fruit
One serving is approximately:
• 1 medium (150g, 5oz) apple, banana, orange or pear
• 2 small (150g, 5oz) apricots, kiwi fruits or plums
• 150g (5oz) of lychees, watermelon, strawberries, blueberries
Palm ≈ 75 grams (3 ounces)
Lean Meats
LM
One serving is approximately:
• 75g (3oz) **low fat** beef, lamb, poultry, fish
• 2 medium eggs
SV
Starchy Veggies
One serving is approximately:
• ½ cup (75g, 3oz) sweet potato, yams, beets, pumpkin, plantains or other **starchy vegetables**
Whole Grains
WG
One serving is approximately:
• 1 (40g, 1.5oz) slice of **bread**
• 2/3 cup (30g, 1.5oz) cereal flakes
• ¼ cup (30g 1.5oz) muesli
• ½ cup (75g, 3oz) **cooked rice**, pasta, noodles, quinoa
FM
Fatty Meats
One serving is approximately:
• 75g (3oz) beef, lamb, poultry, fish with **visible fat**
Cupped hand ≈ ½ cup
Dairy
One serving is approximately:
• 1 cup (250ml) milk
• 2 slices (40g, 1.5oz) **hard cheese**
• ¾ cup (200g, 7oz) yoghurt
• 100g firm tofu
Legumes
One serving is approximately:
• ½ cup (75g, 3oz) **cooked** beans, peas or lentils
Thumb ≈ 30 grams (1 ounce)
Tip ≈ 1 teaspoon
Nuts & Oils
One serving is approximately:
• 30g (1oz) almonds, cashews, macadamia and other **nuts**
• 1 tablespoon (15g, ½oz) coconut oil
Sugar
One serving is approximately:
• 1.5 teaspoons (7g, ¼oz) table **sugar**
• 2 tablespoons (30g, 1oz) xylitol, erythritol and **sweeteners**

THINKLEANMETHOD.com

Come and visit us at

www.**think**leanmethod.com

for more articles and
information to help you succeed!

References:

While creating the Think Lean Method and subsequently writing this book, I focused on peer-reviewed research published in respected journals. This produces high quality results that are supported by evidence.

The majority of studies referenced are freely available online. You can find these by searching for the title of the study, and then following the links to "Free Full Text" where available. Don't be scared to look them up. They are generally easier to read than what you'd think!

---

1 A. Belza, C. Ritz, M.Q. Sørensen et al., "Contribution of gastroenteropancreatic appetite hormones to protein-induced satiety" *American Society for Nutrition*, 2013.

2 D. Yang, Z. Liu, H. Yang et al., "Acute effects of high-protein versus normal-protein isocaloric meals on satiety and ghrelin" *European Journal of Nutrition*, 2013.

3 A. Kozimor, H. Chang, J.A. Cooper, "Effects of dietary fatty acid composition from a high fat meal on satiety," *Appetite*, 69:39-45, Oct 2013.

4 D.K. Layman, E. Evans, J.I. Baum, J. Seyler, D.J. Erickson, R.A. Boileau, "Dietary protein and exercise have additive effects on body composition during weight loss in adult women" *J Nutr*, Aug 2005.O225:O244

5 E. Jequier, "Pathways to obesity." Int J Obes, 2002.

6 O. Oyebode, V. Gordon-Dseagu, A. Walker, J.S. Mindell, "Fruit and vegetable consumption and all-cause, cancer and CVD mortality: analysis of Health Survey for England data" *J Epidemiol Community Health*, March 2014

7 R.J. Wurtman, J.J. Wurtman, "Brain serotonin, carbohydrate-craving, obesity and depression," *Obes Res*, Nov 1995.

8 J.D. Fernstrom, R.J. Wurtman, "Brain serotonin content: increase following ingestion of carbohydrate diet," *Science*, Dec 1971.

9 K.L. Teff, S.S. Elliott, M. Tschöp, T.J. Kieffer, D. Rader, M. Heiman, R.R. Townsend, N.L. Keim, D. D'Alessio, P.J. Havel, "Dietary fructose reduces circulating insulin and leptin, attenuates postprandial suppression of ghrelin, and increases triglycerides in women" *J Clin Endocrinol Metab*, 2004.

10 N.M. Avena, P. Rada, B.G. Hoebel, "Sugar and Fat Bingeing Have Notable Differences in Addictivelike Behavior" *Journal of Nutrition*, March 1, 2009.

11 G. Dimitriadis, P. Mitrou, V. Lambadiari, E. Maratou, S.A. Raptis, "Insulin effects in muscle and adipose tissue" *Diabetes Res Clin Pract*, Aug 2011.

12 R. Koopman, A.J.M. Wagenmakers, R.J.F. Manders, A.H.G. Zorenc, J.M.G. Senden, M. Gorselink, H.A. Keizer, L.J.C. van Loon, "Combined ingestion of protein and free leucine with carbohydrate increases postexercise muscle protein synthesis in vivo in male subjects" *American Journal of Physiology – Endocrinology and Metabolism*, 1 April 2005.

13 B.B. Rasmussen, K.D. Tipton, S.L. Miller, S.E. Wolf, R.R. Wolfe, "An oral essential amino acid-carbohydrate supplement enhances muscle protein anabolism after resistance exercise" *Journal of Applied Physiology*, Feb 2000.

14 M.N. Harvie, M. Pegington, M.P. Mattson, et al., "The effects of intermittent or continuous energy restriction on weight loss and metabolic disease risk markers: a randomised trial in young overweight women" *Int J Obes (Lond),* 35(5): 714–727, May 2011.

15 J.S. Volek, M.J. Sharman, A.L. Gómez, D.A. Judelson, M.R. Rubin et al., "Comparison of energy-restricted very low-carbohydrate and low-fat diets on weight loss and body composition in overweight men and women" *Nutr Metab (Lond),* 1: 13, 2004.

16 A.R. Skov, S. Toubro, B. Rùnn, L. Holm, A Astrup, "Randomized trial on protein vs carbohydrate in ad libitum fat reduced diet for the treatment of obesity," *Int J Obes (Lond),* 23, 528±536, 1999.

17 T.A. Astorino, M.M. Schubert, "Individual responses to completion of short-term and chronic interval training: a retrospective study," *PLoS One*, May 2014.

18 A. Tremblay, J.A. Simoneau, C. Bouchard, "Impact of exercise intensity on body fatness and skeletal muscle metabolism," *Metabolism*, Jul 1994.

19 M.S. Treuth, G.R. Hunter, M. Williams, "Effects of exercise intensity on 24-h energy expenditure and substrate oxidation," *Med Sci Sports Exerc*, Sep 1996.

www.ingramcontent.com/pod-product-compliance
Lightning Source LLC
Chambersburg PA
CBHW051612030426
42334CB00035B/3494

* 9 7 8 0 9 9 4 2 4 1 2 1 4 *